# Introduction To Clinical Effectiveness And Audit In Healthcare

# Introduction To Clinical Effectiveness And Audit In Healthcare

## Dr. PS Reddy

Consultant Child and Adolescent Psychiatrist

**To order additional copies of this book, contact:**

Xlibris Corporation

0-800-644-6988

www.xlibrispublishing.co.uk

Orders@xlibrispublishing.co.uk

303016

# Contents

The central purpose of this handbook is to motivate clinical trainees and professionals involvement in clinical effectiveness and audit. Local small scale audits are the most feasible practical audits for undergraduates and trainees. This book aims to provide a good basic understanding of designing and completing such audits. However an overview of the whole range of possibilities is explained to understand the significance of clinical effectiveness, audit and quality improvement within healthcare organisations.

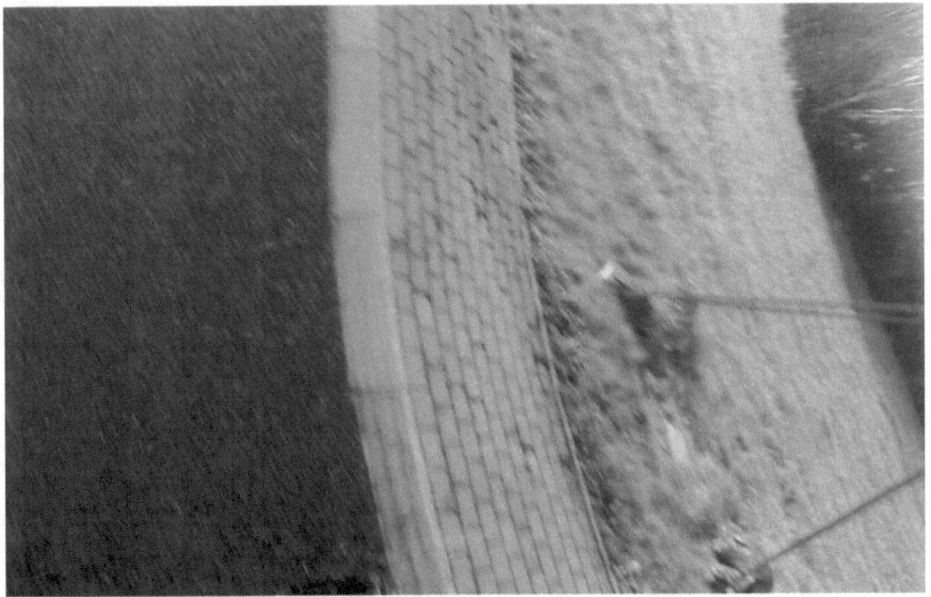

Making things right needs an understanding of the process and structural perspective. Good Intentions need good evidence and effective feedback to recognize and deliver good care.

# Preface

The central purpose of this handbook is to motivate clinical trainees and professionals involved in clinical care about the principles and practice of clinical audit and medical audit in improving clinical effectiveness. Local small scale audits are the most feasible practical audits for undergraduates and trainees. This book aims to provide a basic understanding of designing and completing such audits. However an overview of the whole range of possibilities is explained to understand the significance of the audit exercise within local and national organisations.

The many different models for clinical audit which have been completed at national and local levels are explained. Examples of good practice are an essential part of planning an audit and I sincerely hope that this handbook motivates the trainees and clinical professionals from various specialities to focus on such examples to follow through in future. A practical way of introducing trainees early in the training phase will significantly complement the theoretical knowledge and evidence based and focussed evaluation techniques used in their training and assessments.

An introduction to clinical governance and research has been included to provide an understanding of the role of audit in the general scheme of quality assurance in health care organisations. The evolutionary nature of healthcare service reform and frequent updates in medical technology and research needs a flexible medical workforce which can incorporate and assess changing examples of good practice. Audit is an important method to evaluate the practice and applicability of such good practice examples set by organisations in an objective way.

In the United Kingdom Healthcare reform over the last 2 decades has been centrally driven on an unprecedented scale ever since universal free healthcare was introduced after it became a welfare state in 1948. It has led the world in providing a socialist model of ethical healthcare accessible to all citizens. Various organisations like Healthcare Commission, National Institute for Clinical Excellence (NICE), the Clinical Governance Support Team (CGST) and the National Audit and Governance Group (NAGG) have been contributors for the national strategy for audits.

However the frequent changes in the names and roles of individual organisations with a particular emphasis on strategic flexible management in contrast to the older time focussed planning like five year plans, needs constant updating and continues to change to date. The initial top down nature of these reforms have now been instilled into routine clinical practice and has been a unique management exercise for the government. The closure of the Clinical governance support team has been a significant indicator of such a change especially in England.

I am indebted to all those who have assisted in the development of this handbook. My particular thanks to all members of clinical staff and my family who have given their time, feedback and enthusiasm during the evolution of this book.

Dr PS Reddy

# Introduction

Assessing quality in medicine objectively has historically been a difficult task. Therefore throughout history the focus has been on the quality of the people who deliver it encapsulated by the Hippocratic Oath(1) and later by the World health Organisation in the Geneva Declaration (2). These qualities were later predominantly categorised as ethical issues. Regulatory agencies have selectively names a few of these qualities as competence.

In the past a robust system of intensive training with an equally efficient assessment system were considered enough to maintain high standards of care for the patients. However a few cases of undetected deliberate ethical mistakes have caused significant concern among professionals and patients(3,4). The rising awareness of concerned patients have reflected the governments resolve for quality management in the Health Services (3,4).

Clinical audit was a tool to bring in organisational systemic changes introduced in the United Kingdom. It was formally introduced into the National Health Service in 1993 as a central strategy to reform the organisations quality assurance through Clinical Governance and was defined as "a quality improvement process that seeks to improve patient care and outcomes through systematic review of care against explicit criteria and the implementation of change"(3).

The white paper (1989) 'Working for patients' (5) defined medical audit as "Systematic critical analysis of the quality of medical care including the procedures used for diagnosis and treatment, the use of resources and the resulting outcome and quality of life for the patient."

A variant term Clinical Audit was added with a similar definition "Systematic analysis of the quality of healthcare, including the procedures used for diagnosis, treatment and care, the use of resources and the resulting outcome and quality of life for the patient."

The National Institue of Health and Clinical Excellence in the United Kingdom (NICE) (7) published the paper '*Principles for Best Practice in Clinical Audit*', which defines clinical audit as "a quality improvement process that seeks to improve patient care and outcomes through systematic review of care against explicit criteria and the implementation of change. Aspects of the structure, processes, and outcomes of care are selected and systematically evaluated against explicit criteria. Where indicated, changes are implemented at an individual, team, or service level and further monitoring is used to confirm improvement in healthcare delivery."

The concept of clinical audit covers a wider range of activities compared to the American system of Health Care Effectiveness initiated by Ernest Codman(8) who lost his staff previleges for his plan to evaluate surgical competence.

Various definitions of Audit are in practical use. The most commonly used was the definition provided by the Department of Health(3). However a comprehensive functional definition (Table 1) can encapsulate the core utility of the terms.

Table 1

**Functional Definition**

1. Medical/Clinical audit is an Institutional/organisational quality assessment and improvement process. The distinction between medical and clinical audit was due to professional boundaries rather than any clinical need.

2. It seeks to improve all aspects of patient assessment, care and outcomes through a cyclical process of evaluation, identification of strengths and weaknesses, implementing change, re-evaluation and monitoring change. The aim is to incrementally improve on the quality and focus on indicators that can be changed.

3. It is achieved by a systematic review of standards of individual patient assessments and management of healthcare against explicit evidence based gold standard criteria with an emphasis on systemic and team based performance with no specific focus on individual responsibility.

4. If necessary Implementation of change is through systemic organisational change achieved through feedback in various specifically organised systemic Clinical Governance structures.

5. Further monitoring is used to confirm improvement in healthcare delivery and complete the audit cycle.

6. If the standards are met, planned strategies should continue to monitor any critical incidents that are likely to happen and reauditing needs to be restricted to promote efficacy and should be discouraged if improvement is not likely to be achieved.

7. At the end of the audit certain survey parameters need to be agreed to monitor that outcomes are being met.

## History

Audit is a process involving performance evaluation of a person, team or organization. Audits are performed to ascertain the validity and reliability of information, and also provide an assessment of a system's functioning. which adhere to generally accepted standards set by governing bodies. Such an origin can explain the close relationship between the terms governance and audit within the management structures of Healthcare organisations. There is a significant difference between Clinical Audit and the other forms of audit. Clinical audit process is carried out by healthcare professionals themselves though the burden of required changes does fall on the governing management framework.

The principle of not focussing on individual responsibility is based on risk management principles used in Crew Resource Management, formerly known as Cockpit Resource Management. It has its roots in United Airlines where a formal training programme was set up to concentrate on the human factor in aviation mishaps (10). Communication of errors without fear of being blamed with clear delegation of duties in a team to maximise effectiveness and minimise risks is central to this process.

Systematic Audit in medical science is a relatively new introduction to healthcare. It has its origin from the financial regulation of capitalist institutions. It adds a corrective dimension within the aristocratic sounding Clinical Governance framework of effective management. Though such a negative attitude of high handed regulation has been perceived negatively by critics, it has provided significant opportunities in improving the health care system and is currently widely accepted. Its introduction was piloted on an industrial scale in the United Kingdom healthcare system. It has been a dramatic decade of centrally driven systemic changes in the nationally managed health service which most countries can only aspire to have. The focus has been on different aspects of the system including management and clinical care at all levels of healthcare ranging from a National level, Strategic Health Authorities, Organisations, Divisional and Subdivisional managerial and clinical levels and including Individual teams of professionals both within a particular discipline and as part of multidisciplinary joint work.

Historically in 1750 BC, King Hammurabi (3) of Babylon instigated assessment for clinicians with regard to their patients outcome. Some resulted in serious consequences for the clinician involved even when it was accidental. Functionally however such individual accountabilities are more to do with clinical competence than with an audit and do not seem to contain all the essential components of audit.

More rational and humane audit like assessments were done by Florence Nightingale (3) who audited infection rates in 1856 before and after improving general hygiene. Dr Ernest Cobman (9) evaluated post surgical outcomes in Massachusets Hospital (1914) with individual accountability which was unpopular. However they failed to fulfil all the criteria to meet the definition of medical audit.

Between 1988 to 1990, official systemic funding of audit activity throughout the National Health Service started in the United Kingdom (3). Initially medical care provided by doctors was audited and was termed 'Medical Audit'. It however evolved to encompass all aspects of patient care, and with the involvement of all clinical staff and the term 'Clinical Audit' was introduced.

The introduction of clinical governance into organisations following the publication of the United Kingdom government's White Paper 'The New National health Service, Modern, Dependable' (9) was the next step that made it a statutory duty for all Organisations to ensure quality upon all Health care providing bodies. Clinical audit is a key and essential component of clinical governance. The other aspects of clinical governance are discussed in chapter 2. It provided a framework for organisation and implementation of the audit programme throughout Organisations.

## Structural organisation of Clinical Audit management

All Organisations now have defined responsibilities for clinical audit activity in the United Kingdom. The focus is on Implementing at a local level. The culture of initiation into audit needs to start from initial medical training. A brief guide to the structural organisation and processes necessary to deliver clinical audit at various levels is described in Table 2

Table 2.

| **Organisation of Clinical audit management in Health authorities and Organisations.** |
| --- |
| Within health care the Specialist health care Organisations and General Pactice Clinics are two functionally seperate Health organisations with separate clinical and financial accountability but can be considered to be identically similar since they both provide healthcare at different ends of the spectrum. |
| The clinical governance lead is the responsible person statutorily nominated for clinical audit programmes within local Organisations. In the United Kingdom it is a statutory duty and responsibility. <br><br> There is also a statutory duty for these audits to reflect national audit priorities within the United Kingdom. However a chain of delegations of duties exists depending on size of trusts and resources available. <br><br> Responsibilities for some managers rests in delegating and monitoring and for some in engaging all clinical staff in audits. |
| The nominal head of the organisation along with the medical lead are responsible for the quality of care delivered by any individual Organisations and therefore are considered responsible for clinical audit. Some smaller trusts may only afford to have a single person in both roles. |
| The nominal head of the organisation along with the medical lead may appoint a clinical governance lead to coordinate clinical governance activities including clinical audit. |

The clinical governance lead ultimately retains delegated accountability for clinical audit, but may choose to delegate this role to the clinical audit lead. This chain of beureaucracy helps in providing resources in all levels of management and helps at all strategic levels of planning.

Role of a clinical audit lead includes
1. Coordinating audit programmes at the local level
2. Create a clinical audit strategy based on national and local priorities and capabilities
3. Setting operational audit priorities based on audit strategy
4. Empowering and encouraging clinical members to Implement the strategy and audit programmes by providing resources and expertise
5. Build the network of clinical audit committee
6. Create a culture of openness within institutions where mistakes are discussed and dealt with effectively addressing organisational failures and weaknesses through empowered and proactive healthcare workforce.

## The Clinical Audit Manager

A Clinical Audit Manager refers to a responsible clinical audit staff member who manages a central coordinating role. The strategic plan of audit leads need resources coordinated by the clinical audit manager to operationalise and mediate the interactions with clinical staff doing audits. The role has significant responsibilities but has a potentially important role of coordinating operational resources, identifying important audit subjects and providing the resources and getting things done operationally in the most effective and efficient way. The Clinical Audit Manager is accountable to the clinical audit lead.

The Manager retains overall responsibility for the management of the staffing resource and the allocation of staff. His responsibilities include project managing the resources to deliver the programme developed by Clinical Audit Committee. The main role lies in identifying the statutory role of clinical audit for all staff, make arrangements to have delegated time for all staff to be involved in the process of planning, developing and performing audits. They are also responsible for arranging audit meetings and communicating results of audits to the strategic planning teams to help risk minimisation and efficacy improvement programmes to incorporate audit recommendations. This operational role is considered vital in implementing the clinical audit programme. Most trainees fail to utilise this important resource which can help prevent repeating audits that may not be of any benefit to the organisation.

## Types of Audit Departments

There are two main types of audit departments described within Organisations(3). The Bristol Royal Infirmary Inquiry set up after a investigation of poor cardiac surgeries because of staff resistance to change and to accept modern developments in children's cardiac surgeries (4) recommended a central audit department. However larger organisations need a much devolved system with audit coordinators for different departments. The two main predictors of performance are strategic management leadership and a proactive staff involved multidisciplinary audit programme.

Table 3

| Centralised audit department | Devolved audit department |
|---|---|
| Managers and facilitators sited in one place | Managers are centrally based but facilitators are spread across divisions |
| Suitable for small Organisations | Suitable for large Organisations spread across a wide area |
| Appear detached, formal, out of touch and bureaucratic | More informal, in touch and better coordinated |
| Easy to detach staff from inappropriately engaging in helping out with the audit and focus on better productivity from resources | Staff may be drawn into getting involved in doing the audit rather than coordinating. |
| Easier for Audit Manager to ensure supervision and personal development of audit staff | May be difficult for audit manager to coordinate staff |

## Clinical Audit Patient Panel

Surveys and reports in the past have consistently revealed that patient involvement in delivery of healthcare was not satisfactory. The only way to improve this is by participation of service users in delivering care.

Though there are evidence-based clinical guidelines and National Service Frameworks advocate service users involvement, patients and public expectations have rarely been taken into account. Therefore patient involvement needs to be actively encouraged. However such involvements need to have a specific need and task. Ethical issues with regard to confidentiality should be discussed and if required assessed by the ethics committees.

A logical next step was to create a Clinical Audit Patient Panel (CAPP) (3). They can advise on validity of various audit criteria and ways of assessment that would help in getting an objective result. Though there are provisions for such an arrangements they are uncommonly used. Members can be actively involved in all phases of the audit.

If we aspire to improve services and ensure that patients feel that they have ownership of their care, it is important to ensure that patients remain at the centre of the organisation. They can be empowered through active patient and service use involvement. However when involving patients it must be clear from the very start the reason patient is involved and how they are expected to assist the service. Service users can be genuine collaborators, rather than just being sources of data.

Clinical audit assists and develops services in improving patient care. Therefore it is logical to consider feasibility of creating a Clinical Audit Patient Panel in all possible situations. Involving patients is key to developing services. They can tell us a range of things: how to communicate, how we make them feel, how convenient the service is, how we respect them and their culture, whether we involve them in decisions and whether they trust us.

In spite of our best intentions as service providers evidence and experience from the past suggests we can get it wrong without feedback from service users.

Recent research indicates that a patient is more likely to tell another patient something that they would never mention to their health care provider. Patients referred to out-patient clinics may have misconceptions about what will happen when they attend. Patients' expectations are linked to drop-out rates, satisfaction and outcome(14).

Table 4: Member requirements for Patient or Service User Panel

| |
|---|
| 1. Panel members have a basic knowledge and understanding of clinical audit and therefore, |
| 2. Basic clinical audit training should be |
| 3. A clinical audit guide should also be provided for each panel member. |
| 4. Confidentiality must be ensured by confidentiality agreement approved by the Caldicott Guardian. |
| 5. Issues around staff feeling that they are being criticised/undermined need to be addressed by a policy that patients will not work with their own service that they are currently using. |

## Other non audit clinical activities

There are many activities done in Health care delivery that would not be considered as clinical audit.

**1.** *Routine statistics*

The collection of data not related to clinical standards is not considered to be clinical audit. Preaudit is a term used for data collection only for setting standards of best practice. But this distinction is not very clear and is currently obsolete. It could however be the initial phase of the audit if a good reason exists for the need for completing the audit cycle. Otherwise it would be more appropriate to use the term survey for such an exercise.

Table 4

| |
|---|
| **Sources of routine data** |
| Various sources of routinely collected data are available for use in epidemiological studies. These include: |
|    • Demographic data from census and population registers<br>   • Death certificates after registration<br>   • Cancer and serious illness registrations<br>   • Birth registrations<br>   • Infectious disease notifications<br>   • Hospital episode data and critical incidents<br>   • Health surveys |

## **2**. *Routine Monitoring of Clinical Outcomes*

Routine monitoring of clinical outcomes is part of assessment of quality in any organisation. It is a part of routine surveillance. It can be compared over periods of time for the same proceedure. However it differs from audit by not having specific gold standard measures put in place before reaudits are performed. In addition there is no plan and action about a process to change the next comparable measure. Examples of such surveillance programmes are performance monitoring for professionals and disability or quality of life assessments among patients. The identification and measurement of clinical outcomes may form a significant part of a clinical audit. If such clinical outcomes are already at a nationally expected standard there is very little use in auditing them. However if such a surveillance reveals a standard below what is expected there is a clear need for an audit process.

Routine Outcome Monitoring is an important quality tool for measuring outcome of treatment in health care. The evidence supports a positive impact of monitoring on diagnosis and treatment, and on communication between patient and therapist among adults. Other results are unclear. There were no published Randomised Controlled Trials in children or adolescents. It appears to be especially effective for the monitoring of patients who are not doing well in therapy. It holds true for both physical and mental illness (15).

## **3.** *Peer Review*

The purpose of peer review is to assure that quality controls are being applied in conformity with quality control standards. Peer review has a long history, but quality-improvement techniques for enhancing quality of care initiatives have only been in use for the last two decades. It can be an individuals review or review of similar team based services.

It is currently part of appraisal of professional competence and performance for individual healthcare providers. It involves a similar group of clinicians selecting a small sample of patients recently under their care and collectively considering whether the best possible care was provided or whether things might have been done differently. Such an exercise needs to be meaningful to gain insight into mistakes and not just a post mortem of how the management was completed. Hence it is more of an active process of reflective learning and management where peers are actively consulted for their opinions and if ambivalent issues remain a consensus is reached about management.

Peer review needs to have the following characteristics

## Table 5

---

- Consistent with hospital policy and a consistent standard.
- Needs to be regular and not driven by case volume and conducted monthly or quarterly.
- Objective agreed conclusions set before peer review
- Standards agreed taking national and local parameters.
- Review by comparable peer. A surgeon is not evaluated by a physician, but a peer surgeon.
- Agree on useful action so the physician under review has the opportunity to improve techniques, skills, and abilities to achieve the needed level of competency.
- Regular auditing of process and standards

---

## 4. *Mortality & Morbidity (M&M) reviews*

They are specific kinds of peer reviews. They look at adverse outcomes like death (mortality), disability or disease (morbidity). They are comprehensive investigations of specific cases with adverse outcomes and looking for prevention strategies for similar outcomes in the future. They differ from audit in various ways.

The principal distinction is that these are not planned processes that can be relevantly measured and reaudited. Their nearest audit relative is the critical incident audit. However distictions are clear cut and validated.

The forum for discussion of morbidity and mortality within a department or unit is known by different names: morbidity and mortality review (MMR); morbidity and mortality conference (MMC) and morbidity and mortality meeting (MMM). No functional differences between the three terms exist and they mean the same. The purpose of individual MMRs varies. The most commonly reported goals overall were medical management, teaching, patient safety and quality improvement (16).

## 5. *Significant Event Audit*

These are a type of peer review in primary care with assessment of Identified events looking for information relevant to an adverse or potentially adverse outcome. The purpose is to identify what went wrong, likely causes and remedies. It enables teams to learn from patient safety incidents and 'near misses', and to highlight and learn from both strengths and weaknesses in the care they provide. There are 7 steps described in performing a significant event audit.

Table 6

---

**The seven stages of Significant Event Audits:**

---

- Awareness and prioritisation of a significant event
- Information gathering
- The facilitated team-based meeting
- Analysis of the significant event
- Agree, implement and monitor change
- Write it up
- Report, share and review

---

## 6. *Patient Surveys*

They can constitute research, feedback or audits depending on design.

## 7. *Service evaluation*

Occasionally attempts have been made to evaluate some services with no systematic evidence about outcomes. In such cases the term Service Evaluation has benn used to define "A set of procedures to judge a service's merit by providing a systematic assessment of its aims, objectives, activities, outputs, outcomes and costs" (11)

Evaluation provides practical information to help decide whether a development or service should be continued or not. Evaluation also involves making judgements about the value of what is being evaluated. It is not a way of circumventing the rigid evidence based structural assessments to implement politically driven and consensually agreed services. It is based on empirical evidence of necessity.

Table 7

| Service Evaluation characteristics |
| --- |
| 1. Usually can be designed within an audit framework |
| 2. May provide cost and/or benefit information on a service |
| 3. Uses quantitative and qualitative data to explore activities and issues |
| 4. May identify strengths and weaknesses of services |
| 5. May include elements of research eg collecting additional data or changes to choices of treatment |
| 6. If an evaluation study includes a research project, the research should be managed within the Research Governance Framework. |

## 8. Consensus Methods

It is about agreeing on a method when opinion varies. It has been defined as a process aimed to achieve a result. "The focus of consensus methods lies where unanimity of opinion does not exist owing to a lack of scientific evidence or where there is contradictory evidence on an issue. The methods attempt to assess the extent of agreement (consensus measurement) and to resolve disagreement (consensus development)."(12)

Consensus techniques and consensus workshops are discussion groups involving a communication process used to inform decision-making where evidence is lacking or contradictory. Consensus methods may be used to agree guidelines, priorities, processes or policy. It is based on principles of shared responsibility, evidence evaluation and functionality.

Table 8

| Consensus methods |
|---|
| 1. Delphi method: structured communication technique, originally developed as a systematic, interactive forecasting method which relies on a panel of experts<br>2. Nominal group technique: is a decision making method for use among groups of many sizes, who want to make their decision quickly but need everyone's opinions taken into account without just taking opinion of the majority.<br>3. Consensus conferences. |

Table 9

| Consensus Process: |
|---|
| 1. May involve interviews and/or questionnaires to get explicit opinions<br>2. Those involved are partners rather than participants and their names are usually included in any report or publication for shared responsibility and to validate the process<br>3. May be used to design a research project for controversial issues<br>4. May be used to decide where research is required in prioritising various options given limited resources<br>5. Consensus methods in health care need to keep ethical principles as overriding parameters but would not normally require ethical approval.<br>6. Consensus methods may also form part of a research project and, if so, should be managed as research including getting ethical approval. |

## 9. *Clinical Investigation*

Diagnostic tests as part of clinical investigation is still unclear in a number of illnesses. These may be the subject of a research study especially in situations where diagnosis of disease is difficult. Organisations may request such supportive inconclusive diagnostic tests, in an attempt to support a diagnosis. Where the purpose of requesting the test is to obtain a diagnosis or to determine the appropriate care for a particular patient the request for the test should not be regarded as research. The person requesting the test does not need to be included in an ethics application.

Where the purpose for requesting the test is to help the scientists and researchers in developing a new diagnostic technique, and the aim is to develop the body of knowledge about the technique or the disease, the request for the test should be regarded as part of the research and ethical approval must be sought.(13). In international collaborations, other countries requirements for ethical approval for participating clinicians may be different.

## Research by trainees and students

Student projects in health care need good standards and should be assessed by the same criteria as above and managed as research, where it is research. Sometimes student projects are audits, and in these circumstances, the projects do not need to be managed as research and ethical approval is not required.

### Summary

The terms Clinical Audit and Medical Audit only serve the purpose of professional boundary recognition.

Definitions of audit vary but can be summarised comprehensively as a functional definition.

It can vary in complexity from simple to very complex assessment of quality. But it is a measure of quality rather than quantity. The only limitation in quantity is the numbers required for statistical significance.

It is a statutory duty of all organisations to include audit and prioritise audit topics in the United Kingdom

There is a need for management structure in place to monitor audit in every organisation.

All audits need to be supervised and monitored

A good local environment for audit should be maintained and the health care organisations should make sure that it uses audit outcomes constructively.

Patient involvement is an essential part of audit but needs issues of ethical and confidentiality to be managed effectively.

Clinical audit is different from research. The implications are that resources for research should not be used for audit. However such clear distinctions are unclear in some situations.

There are other routine proceedures to ensure quality which are not to be considered audit though they can be modified to be an audit

## References

1. http://en.wikipedia.org/wiki/Hippocratic_Oath
2. http://en.wikipedia.org/wiki/ Declaration_of_Geneva
3. Clinical Governance Support Team, A Practical Handbook for Clinical Audit. 2004
4. Department of Health. Learning from Bristol: the Report of the Public Inquiry into Children's Heart Surgery at the Bristol Royal Infirmary 1984-1995. Command paper CM 5207. London: The Stationery Office, 2001.
5. Department of Health, Working for patients. London: The Stationery Office, 1989 6. NHS Executive, Promoting clinical effectiveness. A framework for action in and through the NHS. London: NHS Executive, 1996
7. National Institute of Clinical Excellence, Principles of Best Practice in Clinical Audit. London: NICE, 2002.
8. Mallon, Bill (2000). Ernest Amory Codman: The End Result of a Life in Medicine. Philadelphia: WB Saunders.
9. The New NHS, Modern, Dependable, London:HMSO, 1997
10. *http://airlinesafety.com*
11. *"An introduction to service evaluation"*, Royal College of Psychiatrists Research Unit, 1997.
12. J. Jones, D. Hunter; BMJ 1995;311:376-380 *http://bmj.bmjjournals. com/cgi/content/full/311/7001 /376*
13. BMJ    2004;329:624.    http://bmj.bmjjournals.com/cgi/content/full/329/7466/624

14. B. C. Douglas, L. M. Noble and S. P. Newman, Psychiatric Bulletin 1999, 23:425-427. out-patient consultation
15. *Carlier IV, Meuldijk D, Van Vliet IM, Van Fenema E, Van der Wee NJ, Zitman FG.* Routine outcome monitoring and feedback on physical or mental health status: evidence and theory. J Eval Clin Pract. 2010 Sep 16. doi: 10.1111/j.1365-2753
16. *http://www.health.vic.gov.au/clinicalengagement/downloads/ pasp/literature_review_mortality_ and_ morbidity_reviews.pdf*

# Clinical Governance and Research

## Definition

*Governance* is a word derived from Latin that suggests "steering". The term Governance relates to decisions by a specifically structured hierarchy of management in an organisation with regard to a managed situation or personnel that defines expectations, empowers individuals for performing specific tasks and also verifies performance in a time and cost effective manner. It is a term which is historically related to relatively more authoritarian leadership role in management. It is also a term more commonly used in running government policies. In health care organisations it may relate to a more top down way of management (1).

Governance needs to be distinguished from politics. Politics involves processes by which an empowered group of people reach collective decisions and enforce it as common policy. Governance is an administrative implementation. It can be a y logical policy. It involves multiple functions required in managing strategies and implementing operational policies. The implementing body usually is a group of managers with significant authority and can have an impact on the whole organisation.

Clinical Governance is a statutory term closely associated with audit. In more practical usage audit is a part of clinical governance. It forms part of the system for improving the standard of clinical practice. Clinical governance was introduced to meet need for accountability for the safe management of health services within large organisations where risk minimisation cannot be justified nor acceptable and accepted robust policies need to be in place to prevent it.

This was due partly to the public's and professionals' perception of systemic failings within the health care organisations. In addition there has been a rising expectations from the Health services. It is a challenge that health care professionals have successfully incorporated into their routine care quality maintenance and risk management. Regulatory bodies of all clinical specialities now recognise it as part of good practice and it is a widely accepted model of regulation of quality in service delivery.

Clinical Governance is a system through which organisations are accountable for continuously improving the quality of services. This ensures accountability and a comprehensive programme of quality improvement systems which can effectively minimise risks and prevent harmful mistakes. As the definition of governance implies, the government in the United Kingdom planned a coherent group of six processes that keep the system continuously adaptive with an emphasis on quality(1). ( Table 1)

Table 1
The six pillars of clinical governance

| |
|---|
| 1. Clinical Effectiveness |
| 2. Research & Development |
| 3. Openness |
| 4. Risk Management |
| 5. Education & Training |
| 6. Clinical Audit |

The 1997 White Paper, "The New National Health Service, Modern, Dependable", brought together all service improvement processes into Clinical Governance framework(1). The 6 pillars are described as mutually dependant processes. They share some of the same structural components. It has been an evolutionary step in giving structure to a functional concept. However due to the multiplicity of factors this simplistic definition has been criticised as not being fit for purpose. Consequently a whole range of changes have been made to validate the concept and discussed in the evolution of the concept.

## Evolution of the concept

There is no doubt that Clinical governance is a statutory system for improving the standard of clinical practice. The concept was part of the strategic policy approach to "Creating a First Class Service", whose policy aim was "to provide any autonomous health care organisation that continually improve the overall standard of clinical care, while reducing variations in outcomes of, and access to services as well as ensuring that clinical decisions are based on the most up-to-date evidence of what is known to be effective". Clinical governance was first described in a government White Paper as 'a new system in Organisations and primary care to ensure that clinical standards are met, and that processes are in place to ensure continuous improvement, backed by a new statutory duty for quality in Organisations'.(1)

The new framework has developed in 2 different directions

1.  In the initial phase as a statutory requirement all autonomous health care organisation in United Kingdom have implemented the clinical governance programme for quality assurance. This was a centrally driven top down policy.
2.  As the policy has gained ground the central coordinating structures have now been dismantled.

A strategic way of management has resulted in numerous changes of central regulation. Though this has taken a long time to evolve it has recently been taken off the government's centrally driven agenda by closing the **Clinical Governance Support Team (CGST)** in the United Kingdom and delegating the work back to the autonomous Health organisations which themselves have been reorganised.

## The Seven Pillar Model

The pitfalls of the initial simplistic model of Clinical Governance was reviewed in the United Kingdom by the Clinical Governance Support Team in 1999. They modified the pillars of the Clinical Governance Framework and added five foundation stones. The Pillars are still relevant especially since they support the apex of good clinical governance which is the 'partnership' that exists between the individual patient and the relevant professionals when they interact. This realisation marked a significant change from the non professional hierarchial governance method of the six pillar model. The significance of the term clinical was realised and emphasised.

Table 3: Seven Pillars Model

| Five Foundation Stones | Seven Pillars |
|---|---|
| 1. Systems awareness<br>2. Teamwork<br>3. Communication<br>4. Ownership<br>5. Leadership | 1. Clinical effectivess<br>2. Risk Management effectiveness<br>3. Patient experience<br>4. Communication effectiveness<br>5. Resource effectiveness<br>6. Strategic effectiveness<br>7. Learning effectiveness |

Table 4: & pillar model with a foundation and apex

| | |
|---|---|
| *Apex* | *Partnership between patient and therapist* |
| *Pillars* | *Clinical Effectiveness, Risk, patient experience, communication, resource, strategy & Learning* |
| *Foundation* | Systems awareness Teamwork communication Ownership Leadership |

The evidence for the foundation stones comes from Health Care Commission Investigations, Bristol Inquiry and the Victoria Climbié Inquiry (2). They are vital for the pillars to stand and support the apex. It reflects the recognition of managerial responsibility of healthcare organisations that held only clinicians responsible for the mistakes without giving thought to the fact that strategic and operational managerial issues over a period of time resulted in creating an environment of complacency.

The initial specifications of the remit of clinical governance have undergone strategic changes and are now an umbrella term for all issues of care and management in organised health care services. The key components are numerous and not exhaustive and may include 'key components and themes, all of which, when effective, combine to make up good clinical governance'. (Table 4)(2)

The elements have no significant order but each has equal value and importance(2). They are interdependent and mutually reinforcing. It is also a recognition that a term like clinical governance is too difficult to be described as a structural model when its main definition is based on its functional utility. In the absence of a coherent definition examples of what clinical governance is and isn't may be expected to dispel some of the misunderstandings (2) (Table 5).

## Table 5

| |
|---|
| 1.  Patient, Public and Carer Involvement |
| 2.  Strategic Capacity and Capability |
| 3.  Risk Management |
| 4.  Staff Management and Performance |
| 5.  Education, Training and Continuous Professional Development |
| 6.  Clinical Effectiveness |
| 7.  Information Management |
| 8.  Communication |
| 9.  Leadership |
| 10. Team Working |

This method may however may be criticised to make defining clinical governance a futile exercise and question its validity against the general business models of management.

## Table 6

| Clinical Governance is about | Clinical Governance is not |
|---|---|
| Patient safety, involving carers, providing highest quality patient care at all times, lifelong learning for professionals, Collective responsibility including managers, being inclusive of everyone, Recognising staff achievements, Common sense, Access to quality care, anywhere, anytime. | just for clinicians, One person's responsibility, A stand alone function, Box ticking exercise, Waste of time, just improving cost efficiency |

## History Of Quality and Clinical Effectiveness in Health Care

Concern for affordable quality healthcare has been the main motive behind the foundation of the world's most enviable National Health Service in the United Kingdom. Principles of quality management are a key facet to the modernisation of healthcare delivery.

Dr. Robert Maxwell had developed the following six dimensions of quality in 1984(3)

Table 6

| |
|---|
| 1. Accessible—in terms of availability with no regard to physical and financial barriers |
| 2. Equitable across the Country, for all social classes, for all disease groups, age range, ethnicity, sexual orientation and gender. |
| 3. Appropriate in terms of its available location and philosophy of care |
| 4. Effective in terms of access, assessment and management |
| 5. Acceptable by providers and service users |
| 6. Efficient in terms of cost and benefit |

Concern about quality does not replace methodical assessment based on reliable evidence especially in Healthcare. In quality assessment, the emphasis has shifted from looking at end results to the process leading up to the end result. Similarly it has moved from therapeutic outcome to resource utilisation and cost benefit analysis.

This change in America has led to the professional standards review organisations being replaced in most hospitals by a unified quality assurance programme monitored by the Joint Commission on Accreditation of Hospitals.

In 1985 a World Health Organisation (WHO) working party differentiated clinical quality itself and quality assurance.

Table 7

| |
|---|
| **Quality assurance**: |
| 1. Providing objective evidence of effective use of public funds. |
| 2. Management as a tool for problem solving |
| 3. Facilitate innovation in healthcare delivery to improve outcomes and efficiency |
| |
| **Clinical quality** has four aspects: |
| 1. Professional performance |
| 2. Efficiency |
| 3. Risk management |
| 4. Patient satisfaction |

**Avedis Donabedian** was a physician and founder of the study of quality in health care and medical *outcomes research*. Avedis Donabedian has contributed significantly to healthcare quality characteristics and the complexity of its measurement. He described the different measurable components of healthcare quality (4).

Table 8

1. **Structure:** Quality of healthcare assessed by studying settings in which care takes place. This can include facilities and equipment, administrative process, qualifications of staff. A good structure for delivery of healthcare plays an important part

2. **Process:** literally means what is actually done in providing care. For example following protocols and guidelines.

3. **Outcome:** Outcome measures change attributable to the intervention/ care received.

Table 9

| Public concerns about the quality of healthcare have been a combination of |
|---|
| 1. An increasing recognition of the adverse events in health care |
| 2. A rise in consumer expectations of health care |
| 3. Serious service failures that questioned quality of the healthcare system. |
| 4. Doubts about affordability and efficiency |

Investigations into adverse events and serious service failures identified serious systems failures contributing even when unprofessional conduct of individual clinicians were identified. Clinical governance and quality management was seen as an efficient way of managing quality and efficiency throughout organisations to address issues that have an influence on individual clinicians competence in organisations.

Research by the National Clinical Governance Support Teams have shown variable confidence in the various clinical governance systems. Very few organisations had considered it as a core requirement. The Integrated Governance has been set up to rectify this anomaly. This involves clinicians working in groups across all levels of healthcare provision to learn from experiences and near misses.

## Clinical governance and Integrated governance

After having defined clinical governance as a process and not a structure it has been important to establish its usefulness as a concept 'that is fit for purpose'. However a management structure to implement the process of governance is vital. Clinical governance recognises that clinical issues are at the heart of healthcare. Successful implementation of good governance is still elusive for many enterprises. Integrated governance is a term specifically used in the context of United kingdom National Health Service. It aims to combine clinical issues not in isolation but in the context of finance, staffing and other non-clinical risks. It was developed by Michael Deighan and John Bullivant as an approach to simplfying the complex *governance* arrangements (5).

Integrated Governance is the means by which management authorities can be empowered to direct and control organisations more effectively. The aim is for healthcare organisations to demonstrate simplified, transparent, ethically governed, strengthened and streamlined governance arrangements. In addition it focuses on the gap between healthcare and other social services and, over time aims to develop integration between health and related social care organisations. The essential need for quality as the driver of change places Clinical governance central to Integrated governance agenda. Integrated governance recognises the dynamic tension of competing elements: national vs local and quality vs cost.

The focus of Integrated clinical governance is on ten improvement activities ( Table 10)

---

- Establish clarity of purpose and strategic objectives of the organisation
- Establish a strategic *annual cycle* of *business* integrating clinical, finance and other parameters
- Ensure integrated quality assurance and financial plan systems are in place
- Take decisions supported by intelligent information
- Create a *committee structure* streamlined with clear terms of reference, delegation and reporting arrangements
- Strengthen audit committee to scrutinise all important activities
- Establish effective financial and clinical supports for the Management Board
- Have a process to ensure Board is fit for purpose through selection, induction,training and frequently review Board members competence
- Agree and apply Board etiquette by consensus. Board members have the responsibility of making decisions for an entire organisation. Sometimes the stress of the job overrides the decorum that many people expect from a board member. Egos can flare and make a board meeting more of a circus than a formal meeting. Board member etiquette not only keeps the meeting on track. It also ensures that all legal and ethical standards are adhered to during and outside the meeting.(6)
- Develop individual *executive* and non-executive directors to ensure board corporacy. The true meaning of corporacy eludes many dictionaries. The literal meaning of 'corporacy may be oversimplified so as to mean that all sites operate in exactly the same way as directed by senior management' It is a term used as a contrast to democracy. (use of such words may defeat the aim of needing to be transparent unless) (7).

---

## Clinical Governance documents published by Department of Health in the United Kingdom

## Table 11

1997–"The New National Health Service Modern, Dependable".

1998–Clinical Governance first defined in the Consultation document, "A First Class Service: Quality in the New National Health Service"

1999–The Health Act 1999 made 'quality' a legal duty.

2000-
1. "The National Health Service Plan"
2. Dept of Health Report: "An organisation with a memory" published report of an expert group on learning from adverse events in the National Health Service

2001-
1. "Learning from Bristol: the report of the public inquiry into children's heart surgery at the Bristol Royal Infirmary" 1984-1995 (The Kennedy Report).
2. "Building a safer National Health Service for patients–implementing an organisation with a memory".

2003-
1. National Audit Office report, "Achieving Improvements through Clinical Governance–A Progress Report on Implementation by Organisations"
2. The Victoria Climbié Inquiry Report

2004-
1. "Standards for Better Health"
2. "The National Health Service Improvement Plan"

2005-
1. National Audit Office Report : "A Safer Place for Patients: Learning to improve patient safety"
2. Publication of "Creating a Patient-led National Health Service: Delivering the National Health Service Improvement Plan"

3. Sixth and final report of the Shipman Inquiry into the criminal conduct of General Practitioner Harold Shipman.

2006–"Good doctors, safer patients": To improve the performance of doctors and to protect the safety of patients

2007-

1. "Trust, Assurance and Safety–The Regulation of Health Professionals in the 21st Century" (Department of Health White Paper).
2. "Safeguarding patients"–Government's response to the recommendations of the Shipman's Inquiry's fifth report and to the recommendations of the Ayling, Neale & Kerr/Haslam Inquiries.
3. "Learning from tragedy, keeping patients safe"–
4. National Audit Office report, "Improving Quality and Safety. Progress in Implementing Clinical Governance in Primary Care: Lessons for the New Primary Care Trusts"

# Measurement of Clinical Governance

Though Clinical Governance has a structure and process the evidence base for governance style of management needs evaluation. In most organisations these are currently numerical values of critical incidents, complaints, compliance with national targets and audits that are the prominent indicators of effective governance.

Over the last decade, several efforts have been made in measuring governance in the international development community to assess and measure the quality of governance of countries all around the world. The most recognised measure comparable internationally has been developed by the world bank with governance issues in sub national level currently being investigated with a specific aim of fighting corruption. However this model may not be suitable for measuring efficacy of clinical governance which has a more flexible approach to management and focusses on continuous development compared to simple governance. Ways of auditing different structures of the health service governanceand clinical services is the focus of this book.

# Research

Clinical Governance strategists have actively tried to differentiate whether projects should be managed within the Research Governance Framework. The main theoretical reasons for such a classification are explained in Table 11.

## Table 12

| |
|---|
| 1. An attempt to differentiate the resources allocated to research diverting to audit which was given high priority by the government |
| 2. To clarify the role of audit |
| 3. As an aid to propogate audit as an exercise of comparable status to research |
| 4. To emphasise that ethics committee approval is not necessary for audits. |

Research can be defined as the 'attempt to derive generalisable new knowledge by addressing clearly defined questions with systematic and rigorous methods'(8).

"Research is concerned with discovering the right thing to do; audit with ensuring that it is done right"(9).

Research and audit projects may look very similar. The basic differences are in their functionality,aims and utility rather than design or structure. Research may examine assessment and prognosis of a illness and outcomes of a particular form of treatment compared to a gold standard. The new method could be better than the gold standard. A Clinical Audit project might be designed in a similar way but the purpose is to see if an assessment ot treatment is being followed as it should be based on current standards and if outcomes reflect such a practice.

However grey areas continue to persist. Clinical Governance within healthcare organisations has a responsibility for assuring the quality of all work undertaken within the service. But innovative work is not necessarily research all the time. Such grey areas where it is not easy to distinguish research from other forms of innovative work needs to be managed ethically and economically through ethics committees and clinical governance processes. Therefore health organisation research and development departments are managed as part of overall clinical governance management to establish such links to clarify issues and responsibilities. If a project seems difficult to categorise, the aims of the project should be assessed and an appropriate audit or research project should be designed to suit the needs. Similarities between audit and research are summarised in Table 12

## Table 13 : Similarities between Research and Audit

1. Both aim to answer a specific question relating to quality of care.
2. Both can be retrospective or prospective.
3. Both involve sampling, questionnaire design and analysis of findings
4. Both can be carried out in large and small scales

Research has always enjoyed a very special place in science but it is not just a scientific method. A broad definition includes 'All activities based on intellectual application in the investigation of matter'. Applied research involves discovering, interpreting, and the development of methods and systems for the advancement of human knowledge on a wide variety of matters. Research can use the scientific method but need not do so.

Scientific research relies on the application of the scientific method. It manipulates inherent curiosity eloquently described as why, what and how. This initial cognitive recognition leads on to a logical series of steps including formulating a hypothesis, testing it out using a variety of methods to establish its validaty and later reliability. Scientific research can be subdivided into different classifications. It its broadest sense a lot of methods used in audit and research are similar

There are elaborate descriptions of differences between clinical audit and research and these are summarised in table 13.

## Table 14

| Clinical Research | Clinical Audit |
|---|---|
| Derived for<br><br>1. The purpose of enquiry<br>2. For new knowledge<br>3. Potentially generalisable<br>4. What is best practice/ is there a better way?<br>5. How good is the treatment or practice compared to gold standard | Derived for<br><br>1. The purpose of quality assurance–to improve<br>2. Patient outcomes by improving professional practice<br>3. Practically generalised<br>4. Is best practice being followed?<br>5. Are we achieving or missing the Gold standard targets |
| Done by research staff<br>May involve new treatments or practice | Done by clinical staff<br>Involves only established treatments and practices |
| Aims of Reseach<br><br>1. Research is a designed process to check validity or develop a hypothesis.<br>2. Research is an investigation about unknown consequences of manipulating variables<br>3. Systematic assessment of qualitative or quantitative opinions, experiences or outcomes of research participants. | Aims of Audit<br><br>Clinical Audit is directly related to improving services against a standard that has already been set by examining:<br>1. Whether or not what ought to be happening is happening<br>2. Whether current practice meets required standards<br>3. Whether current practice follows published guidelines<br>4. Whether clinical practice is applying the knowledge that has been gained through research<br>5. Whether current evidence is being applied in a given situation |

| Methodology | Methodology |
|---|---|
| 1. Research needs to have a design so that it can be replicated to check reliability. | 1. May or may not involve patient contact but generally does not involve disturbance beyond that required for normal clinical management |
| 2. May test a new practice, therapy or drug | 2. Some audits can potentially require substantial patient/carer input and carry risks of distress and psychological harm |
| 3. May involve contact with participants | |
| 4. May involve experiments on human subjects, whether patients, patients as volunteers, or healthy volunteers | 3. Participants are never randomised. Participants may receive different treatments or services but allocation of participants to different groups is through normal clinical decision-making processes |
| 5. May be invasive | |
| 6. May involve collecting data from medical records | 4. Results are not transferable to other settings |
| 7. May solely involve collecting data from medical records | 5. May use research methodologies eg interviews, statistical analysis |
| 8. May involve examining tissue or body samples | 6. Standards of good practice are basis of measurement not hypotheses and/or |
| 9. May involve extra disturbance or work beyond that required for normal clinical | |
| **Sample** | **Sample** |
| 1. Usually involves well-defined, often strict selection criteria for the sample selected | 1. statistical sample calculations and statistical sampling methods may not be applicable though it is recommended. |
| 2. In quantitative research, the sample size is usually defined by statistical methods. In qualitative research,. | 2. There should however be a clear description of how the sample will be obtained and the selection criteria to be used |
| 3. May use interviews or questionnaires | |
| 4. Participants may be randomised | 3. Use preagreed checklists |
| 5. It is intended to publish and disseminate the results beyond the organisation, generally at conferences or in academic journals | 4. Participants may not be randomised |
| | 5. It is intended to disseminate the results and implement changes within the organisation, |
| 6. The results may change practice if new interventions or tests are shown to be effective | 6. The results may change practice if standards are not being maintained. |
| 7. May use controls and placebo | 7. Comparision is with gold standards |

| | |
|---|---|
| Statistics<br>Usually involves statistical analysis to extrapolate from the sample to a wider population. | Usually involves statistical analysis to extrapolate from the sample to a wider population within the same context. |
| Results<br>Clinical research outcome is improved knowledge. | Clinical audit outcome is improved quality of practice; |
| Discussion<br>Comply with research governance<br>Ethics approval | Action points can be formulated<br>Audit cycle needs to be reported to audit department<br>Ethical scrutiny necessary but no need for ethics approval |

## Summary

1. Clinical Governance is an overarching framework of improving and maintaining quality in Healthcare delivery. Defining its structure and process may not be an ideal way to understand it.
2. Integrated governance is a term specifically used in the context of United kingdom National Health Service. It aims to combine clinical issues not in isolation but in the context of finance, staffing and other non-clinical risks.
3. There are differences between audits and Research. Clarity about the boundaries can help in identifying separate resources for both audit and research which are covered under clinical governance.
4. Surveys can be research or audits depending on design.

1. The New NHS, Modern, Dependable, London:HMSO, 1997,
2. http://www.cgsupport.nhs.uk/About_CG/default.asp
3. Maxwell RJ, Quality assessment in health. *BMJ* 1984; 288 doi: 10.1136/bmj.288.6428.1470
4a. Donabedian A. Explorations in quality assessment and monitoring. Vol. I. 4b. The definition of quality and approaches to its assessment, 1980; Vol. II. 4c.The criteria and standards of quality, 1982; Vol. III. 4d.The methods and findings of quality assessment and monitoring: an illustrated analysis. Ann Arbor: Health Administration Press, 1985
5. Andrew Corbett-Nolan, Integrated Governance Toolkit, Health and Social Care Quality Centre, July 2005
6. *http://robertsrules.com/inbrief.html*
7. Lucy Kellaway, ITI bulletin September-October 2003,10-14.

8.  Standards and systems for assuring the quality of innovative work in non-research contexts." Research Governance Framework for Health and Social Care, draft second edition, Autumn 2003 http://www.dh.gov.uk/assetRoot/04/02/08/96/04020896.doc

9.  Smith R. Audit & Research. BMJ 1992; 305: 905-6

# The Audit Cycle

Audits in routine professional business is about checking the robust regulatory mechanisms of an institution and is a one off assessment by an external agency. Clinical audit differes from such audits in different ways.

One such difference is its usefulness as a reevaluation tool, sometimes described as an audit cycle. It is not a regulatory exercise but helps identify self evaluated weaknesses in the process of care delivery to service users preventing delivery of effective services. Clinical Effectiveness however is defined by various methods. The various methods used in effectiveness are generally regarded as evidence based. However various other factors play a role and are summarised in table 1.

Table 1: Factors in evaluating effectiveness of a system

| |
| --- |
| 1. Research Evidence |
| 2. Economic viability |
| 3. Common sense |
| 4. Cultural appropriateness |
| 5. Ethical issues |
| 6. Consent issues |
| 7. Service delivery potential—manpower |
| 8. Measurability |
| 9. Appropriateness |
| 10. Preventive strategies |

An audit cycle inherently implies the need to repeat evaluation after a period of corporate change in service delivery in response to an initial audit. It tests flexibility of the management system and measures for change by reauditing relevant parameters. Such a cycle involving atleast two measures of previously identified relevant parameters separated by a period of improvement in services provided is called an Audit Cycle. Various difficulties exist in realising this process as a valid method since it is a corporate change and needs management processes that are dynamic. The factors that need to be taken into account are summarised in Table 2

## Table 2

1. Top down management model
2. Series of delegations
3. No specified role for the delegators in implementing changes
4. No accountability by delegators
5. Seperation of clinical audit staff from those in management implementing changes

An understanding of the various stages of audit cycle and identifying facilitatory structures and processes is vital in carrying out an audit. Such endeavours need to be carefully supervised at each stage. However they should not just be an educational issue for trainees in a team, which is quite often the case. Experienced staff need to be involved in audits themselves and be positive role models. Such modelling provides motivation and the much needed inertia required in large institutions to bring in responsive positive changes in response to audit outcomes.

Though the clinical governance lead is responsible for assuring that there is a clinical audit programme within local trusts their involvement and motivation by attending regular audit meetings is not a requirement. Their involvement in audit is expected to be delegation and they must enforce national audit priorities. Such highhanded authoritarian chain of delegations may sometimes discourage others and this needs to be addressed within the clinical governance framework by delegating explicit responsibilities.

The clinical governance lead ultimately retains accountability for clinical audit, but may choose to delegate this role to another, the clinical audit lead. At a local level this individual will then be responsible for creating a clinical audit strategy, setting audit priorities, agreeing the audit programme, implementing the strategy and implementing the audit programme. The clinical governance lead however retains responsibility for ensuring that these tasks are operationally completed and that clinical audit remains integrated with the other aspects of clinical governance.

The clinical audit lead has a clear role in creating the strategy for embedding clinical audit within the organisation, but the individual or team chosen to perform the audit must have more than just a nominal strategic role. The clinical audit lead should have a high profile within the organisation, and must champion clinical audit both to colleagues and management alike. They should be actively involved in linkages to the other aspects of clinical governance to allow for the dissemination of clinical audit information and the setting of local clinical audit priorities in conjunction with clinicians.

## Clinical audit–the process

Clinical audit can be described as a cycle. Within the cycle there are stages that are expected to follow a systematic process. These include

Table 3

| |
|---|
| 1. Establishing best practice; |
| 2. Measuring against criteria; |
| 3. Action to improve care; |
| 4. Monitoring to sustain improvement |

As the process continues in cycles, each cycle aspires to achieve a higher level of quality.

### 1. Topics and Standards for audit

There are various resources already available readily as topics and gold standards to compare performance. Table 3 summarises these factors

Table 3

| |
|---|
| 1.  National Clinical audit topics take priority |
| 2.  Should be a planned sequence of audits |
| 3.  Should be flexible enough to engage new ideas and to persue subjects of interest |
| 4.  Service users need to be included wherever possible |
| 5.  Critical incidents |

6.  High volume, high risk, high profile and high cost.

7.  Areas where care is recognised to be weak

8.  Subjects of interest to clinical staff

9.  Availability of standards to compare

10. If standards need to be 100% compliant it may not allways be useful to audit them since they are likely to be complied with if adequate safeguards are in place.

11. Should be multidisciplinary in nature.

12. Clinical audit should include assessment of process and outcome of care

## 2. Steps in planning audits

A few logical practical steps in planning successful audits is summarised in table 4. These follow the initial step of selecting audit topic and agreeing standards. This process is best completed within a team with delegated responsibilities agreed beforehand in a planned way. The plan needs to include resources for ensuring audit cycle is completed if required in the future. It may be helpful to review previous audits completed within the organisation and other similar audits completed by other organisations.

## Table 4

1.  Preperation with regard to job plan arrangements, resource allocation and delegated responsibilities.

2.  Literature search to look for other similar audits, acceptable levels of outcomes and in planning resources

3.  Discussion needs to include clinicians and managers

4.  Designing Audit proforma needs a comprehensive review to suit local needs and priorities.

5.  It is recommended to use explicit categorical and unambiguous criteria for aud. The most common acceptable standard is a yes/no response. Likert scales may not be easy to interpret and replicate to compare during audit cycles.

6.  It is very important to ensure Content Validity of the questionnaire. The questions should measure what is intended to be measured.

7.  Sampling method and size—should be adequate to produce credible results. Further information is provided on the section of statistics

8.  Ways of Collecting data ensuring appropriate sampling techniques.

9.  Managers and local leads should be actively involved in audit and the development of action plans
9.  Action plans should not just address the ways forward but address the local barriers to change and delegate the task by identifying those managers and clinicians responsible for service improvement
10. Re-audit should be planned and completed to ascertain whether improvements in care have been implemented as a result of clinical audit.
11. Monitoring systems, structures and specific mechanisms should be made available to monitor service improvements once the audit cycle has been completed.
12. Each audit should have a local lead to ensure quality and supervision.

## Process of clinical audit

### 1. Identify the issue

Selection of a suitable topic needs to balance service needs and interests of auditing personnel. Generally the audit is likely to involve numerical categorical measures of adherence to healthcare processes that have evidence of producing best outcomes for clients. Most audits are for outcomes where national standards and guidelines already exist. In these circumstances there is a likelihood of conclusive evidence about effective clinical practice. Other important issues relate to common problems encountered in clinical practice, patient complaints and concerns about services, poor outcomes identified in routine data collection and service areas of high volume, high risk or high cost.

### 2. Defining standards

Audit criteria refer to categorical explicit statements reflecting standards of service. They define what is being measured objectively. The preset standards of care define the specific aspects of care to be measured, and should always be based on the best available evidence. Some of these are accepted standards across the country and some are applicable locally. It may be helpful to clarify the difference between criteria and standard.

A criteria is a measurable parameter of clinical care or a standard of clinical practice. A standard is a preset threshold of the expected compliance for each criteria usually expressed as a percentage.

*Dr. PS Reddy*

### 3. Collecting data

Data collection needs to be precise and relevant to what is being assessed over a relevant period of previously agreed period of time.Ethical issues must be considered if there are valid concerns about confidentiality and consent. The data collected must relate only to the objectives of the audit.

### 4. Analysis

Results of the data collection need to be compared with agreed criteria and standards. It needs to provide information about standards that were met and, if not, to identify reasons. why the standards weren't met in all cases. In some cases with serious consequences it is important to achieve 100% compliance, in other areas lower compliance levels may be acceptable.

### 5. Stage of improving performace.

After publishing results it is important to discuss it in peer reviews and clinical audit meetings and agree on explicit recommendations for change. Action plans to record recommendations is considered good practice and this needs to include barriers for change and delegated responsibilities with time limits. It may also involve refining audit tool if required.

### 6. Completing the audit cycle:

After an agreed period, audits should be repeated to monitor the dynamic impacts of clinical governance in implementing evidence based changes. It is imports to replicate same strategies for sample collection, methods and data analysis. This makes it comparable with the initial audit. The re-audit should ideally demonstrate that the changes have been implemented and that improvements have been made. Additional re-audits may be necessary. This is a very important step in the process since it measures the operational functionality of the clinical governance structure. Results need to be shared locally and if appropriate widely.

In summary the component parts of Clinical Audit are:

## Table 5

Identifying issues and setting standards

Measuring current practice against evidence based accepted standard outcomes

Comparing results with standards and working out the reasons

Consider effective ways of changing clinical practice re-auditing to make sure practice has improved

The whole process is known as the **audit cycle.**

## Audit and Multidisciplinary teams

The Department of Health in the United Kingdom advises a minimum of 10% of audits across service providers, 30% of audits to be involving multiple services and 50% of audits to be multi professional(1).

All national and local clinical audits should have an identified lead. If the data collection needs resources the clinical audit lead should seek on that individual's behalf contractual time for such work and also offer supervision. Ideally all staff involved in the delivery of clinical care should participate in clinical audit. This includes frontline clinical staff members and trainees and managerial staff.

Organisations have a duty to ensure that there is an identifiable budget for clinical audit including the necessary staff costs. Medical staff are often allocated time within their contracts for audit activity. However medical students may significantly benefit both in terms of knowledge about the subject and about practical clinical experience(2).

## Writing up audit reports

After completing audits it would be useful to write it up clearly to help others use data and also to replicate it if required. Powerpoints are good for presentations and word formats are useful for audit submissions locally and for publications. The component parts of such a report needs to include

## Table 6

1) A title
2) Date of report and duration of audit period and audit cycle
3) Name, department and job title of author—people may wish to contact you about the audit
4) Explain the need for the subject audited
5) Give the criteria and standards that are being used
6) Explain methodology with sufficient information for any person reading your report to understand what you have done, and if need be, to repeat the audit.
7) Results and a summary of important issues.

## Summary

Audit is quality improvement process and therefore should start from known structures or processes that need rectifying.

Such a process in a complex clinical environment needs careful evaluation without resorting to blame and promote openness to confront deficits in care and acknowledgement of need to change.

An intial stage in the audit process is to evaluate outcomes of such standards and see if the measured outcomes are comparable to nationally accepted standards.

The second phase lies in evaluating the outcome of the initial part of the audit to explicitly identify problems.

Such outcomes need to be discussed in a audit discussion forum and an action plan should be developed to improve care.

The action plans need to can be a varied number of interventions.

1. Improvement of policies and protocols—For example prescribing guidelines for sedatives
2. Improvement of concordance with protocols
3. Clinical resources to reduce complications and reduce morbidity and mortality.
4. Refinement of the audit tool or adding new outcome measures if required.
5. Include a review date and delegate tasks to people responsible for their implementation.

The third phase includes a reaudit to demonstrate any changes and to complete the audit cycle. If improvements are of an acceptable standard a sustainable monitoring plan needs to be put in place. Results of all audits should be disseminated locally and nationally if possible.

# References

1. http://www.wales.nhs.uk/sites3/Documents/501/Practical_Clinical_Audit_Handbook_v1_1.pdf
2. Department of Health. Learning from Bristol: the Report of the Public Inquiry into Children's Heart Surgery at the Bristol Royal Infirmary 1984-1995. Command paper CM 5207. London: The Stationery Office, 2001.

# Audit in Preventive Interventions

Preventive Medicine is the care and measures taken to prevent illness in healthy individuals. People at risk are prioritised to drive cost efficiency. Professional preventive care includes examinations and screening tests tailored to meet individual patient's needs. Immunization is a common but important example of preventive medicine.

Good hygiene practices are another essential part of preventive care and health maintenance. Hand washing and bathing are important to cleanse the body of infectious agents. Audits in preventive medicine may include

Table 1

| |
|---|
| 1. Process of measuring standards of identifying at risk individuals |
| 2. Process of using specific screening techniques to for individual groups of people |

## Screening

Screening is a process of identifying apparently healthy people who may be at increased risk of a disease or condition. They can then be offered information, further tests and appropriate treatment to reduce their risk and/ or any complications arising from the disease or condition. One particular way of screening and early intervention is in identification of subclinical disorders.

**Table 2: Audit standards for screening Clostridium deficile in hospital admissions**

1. Staff check for Common clinical features in all vulnerable patients admitted
2. Incidence in at risk groups monitored regularly
3. Causative organism looked for in appropriate samples
4. Laboratory identification confirmation required when appropriate
5. Reservoirs of human importance identified and monitored regularly
6. Transmission and staff hygiene monitored regularly
7. Surveillance policy is in place
8. Policy for methods of control including prevention, response to sporadic cases and outbreak control in place

Auditing in illness prevention usually involves preventive strategies and may not be utilitarian for audits. However an attempt has been made to clarify the nature of risk factors and subclinical symptoms and syndromes to help understand the concept.

## Subclinical disorders and risk factors

Research into so-called 'minor' forms of illnesses and identified risk factors has moved beyond efforts justifying these entities. Though their validity remains questionable they provide important insights into etiopathogenesis and epidemiological factors in both clinical and community populations. The continuous variability in severity of symptoms is currently used to categorically classify current risk factors and subclinical illnesses or disorders based on available evidence.

Current research has focussed on validity of assessment using biological parameters, diagnostic tests and measuring scales standardised for normal and clinical populations. Commonly used screening instruments focus on identifying presence of social and functional disability associated with categorised risk factors or subclinicallt diagnosable conditions or disorders. More recent assessment scales have been developed to help in the exploration of the impact of Subclinical disorders on health, quality of life, and as a predisposing factor for more severe disorders.

As with identified illnesses, pharmacological and psychosocial interventions may be useful treatments in minimizing risk factors. Researchers have begun to examine the nature of such risk factors and milder form of spectrum disorders in specific populations, such as the children, elderly and the medically ill.

## Introduction

Research into sub-threshold forms of illnesses including psychiatric disorders is a relatively new but fast-growing area of study in medicine. The origin of this concept is unclear though it is generally believed to be a term borrowed from medical epidemiological descriptions and later use as a descriptive prefix for covert hypothyroidism. However its contribution to risk factors and subclinical forms of illnesses have been slowly increasing, raising awareness of presence of sub clinical symptom clusters, highlighting problems in current diagnostic classifications, providing insights into role of etiopathogenic factors and epidemiology and providing opportunities to study potential primary prevention strategies in medicine. The most recognisable contribution however has been in family and genetic studies of conditions providing opportunities to study phenotypes and genotypes to infer genetic and environmental influences on etiology.

## Nomenclature

Various terms have been used to describe sub clinical syndromes. The main ones include minor disorder, subsyndromal disorders, spectrum disorders, Subclinical syndromes and borderline disorders. Generally this term implies an illness preceeding onset of a clinicallt recognisable disorder, but recent research has focussed on sub clinical symptoms persistent among patients under remission from illnesses which raises concerns about the need to treat these symptoms like an illness or let them persist until they become clinically significant. Such questions have raised concerns about treating hyperlipidaemia and other risk factors more proactively. Such a predicament is not restricted only to physical illnesses and has been observed in people with psychiatric illnesses like Scizophrenia, Depression and Bipolar disorder.

The terminology of sub clinical syndrome may be an alternative to the confusing terminology since it signifies a group of characterised symptoms, and makes no presumptions about being a disorder. It could however contribute to disorders which may manifest in multisystemic ways. It also can be useful in formulating its etiopathological role and serve as a discrete variable available for manipulation for modifying course and prognosis of any associated disorder.

The different meanings of the term sub clinical syndromes makes it difficult to define. The approach best suited to describe it could perhaps be a functional set of criteria that could help in clarifying the clinical utility of the concept of the term which includes:

Table 3

| |
|---|
| 1. Denote a reliably identifiable phenotype in the population |
| 2. Predict long term outcome |
| 3. Present syndromal symptom cluster |
| 4. Validated by longitudinal studies |

These seem similar to Robins and Guze (1970)(1) Criteria which continues to be the Gold standard for categorical diagnoses. It remains a standard approach for determining diagnostic validity for competing hypothesis and uses data from several domains of enquiry. These include

Table 4

| |
|---|
| 1. Clinicoepidemiological |
| 2. Follow up |
| 3. Family and laboratory studies |

However some differences between a clinically diagnosable disorder from sub clinical disorder is necessary to differentiate the functional use of these terms in clinical practice. In most cases symptom severity is probably the most reliable differentiating factor. Current assessment scales have provided opportunities to have replicable cut off points to make such categorical differentiation valid.

The issues in exploring the relationship between sub clinical syndromes and clinical disorders include the following

Table 5

1. Overlap of operational diagnostic criteria
2. Variation in diagnostic instruments and interpretation of diagnostic criteria
3. Lack of developmental perspective
4 Relative paucity of studies simultaneously examining sub clinical syndromes and psychiatric disorders longitudinally.

With these limitations the following possibilities need to be explored to evaluate relationship between sub clinical syndromes and clinical disorders

Table 6

1. The possibility of sub clinical syndromes and clinical disorders being two distinct and unrelated disorders
2. Developmentally different manifestations of the same disorder
3. A complex relationship lying between these possibilities as suggested by phenomenological and family studies.

## Aetiology

A cause effect relationship of subclinical syndromes to clinical disorders would be an ideal way of explaining the importance of identifying sub clinical disorders. Studies in common psychiatric disorders including schizophrenia and depression support this association This relationship however remains far from conclusive due to a number of reasons. There are multiple pathways to the onset of disorders in adults and there is every reason to believe that the same is true for psychiatric disorders across the lifespan (2). Moreover, there are numerous aetiological theories to account for disorders including genetic, biochemical and endocrine, psychological, social and socio-economic.

In Psychiatry Basic psychopathology remains the cornerstone of psychiatric diagnosis. Psychiatric epidemiology based on phenomenological descriptions and diagnosis has played a crucial role in identifying and generalising the clinical presentations to general populations. But current knowledge of psychopathology and epidemiology need to be much more reliable and valid. In addition sensitivity and specificity factors based on differing criteria for diagnoses pose significant restrictions on associative interpretations.

A longstanding dichotomy of organic and functional diagnosis distinction has been rejected in favour of a more widely acceptable stress vulnerability model in the etiopathogenesis of most psychiatric disorders. Despite considerable advances in psychology and biology the contributions of various psycho biosocial factors for most psychiatric disorders remain far from conclusive. The 'Stress-Vulnerability' model presents a pragmatic model of etiology integrating the various theories (2) and has broad clinical utility.

Confounding factors that may suggest an apparent association between sub clinical syndromes and clinical disorders can blur. These include

Table 7

| |
|---|
| 1. co morbidity |
| 2. Heterogeneity |
| 3. Diagnostic overlap |
| 4. Substance misuse |
| 5. Temporal association |
| 6. Personality factors |
| 7. Social factors |
| 8. Psychological factors |

## Barriers in Clinical audit for subclinical disorders

1. Nice guidelines are increasingly recognised as representing the optimum care standards in terms od management of psychiatric conditions. However there are no guidelines for prevention or management of sub clinical syndromes.
2. Management of sub clinical disorders have very few randomised clinical evidence outcome studies to validate effectiveness. However absence of empirical evidence for the effectiveness of a particular intervention is not the same as evidence for ineffectiveness.
3. Evidence-based treatments are often delivered within the context of an overall treatment programme including a range of activities, the purpose of which may be to help engage the patient, and provide

an appropriate context for the delivery of specific interventions. It is important to maintain and enhance the primary service context in which these interventions are delivered, otherwise the specific benefits of cost effectiveness and service planning will be lost.

4.  Difficulties in validity of diagnosis and variable course of sub clinical syndromes have limited the information on course and outcome. However studies on epidemiology, primary interventional prevention programmes and cost effectiveness evaluations provide some evidence regarding course and prognosis.

5.  The effect of sub clinical states coexisting with medical conditions are unclear and further evidence is required to validate such reports.

6.  Prevention has been traditionally divided into three types: primary, secondary, and tertiary prevention. Due to the unclear division between prevention and treatment these classifications have been viewed as problematic and have been replaced with a new classification system that differentiates among prevention, treatment, and maintenance interventions.

7.  The term, prevention intervention, describes all interventions that take place before the first symptoms of a disorder appear. A treatment intervention is an intervention that is initiated during an active psychological disorder, and maintenance interventions include aftercare and relapse prevention programs.

## Summary

1.  Systems of classification are fundamental to all sciences.

2.  The necessity of classification is to provide a conceptual framework within which to place what is observed, to communicate efficiently about illness states, to allow clarity in diagnosis and management and to predict outcomes to measure change.

3.  Current medical diagnostic systems are predominantly open systems of hypothetical compound constructs which allow meaningful research questions to be posed, the answers to which in turn affect the diagnostic system.

4.  The natural history of sub-threshold conditions remains a matter for further research.

5.  Auditing prevention procedures are difficult in view of the scale of the at risk population and the absence of clinical symptoms

# References

1.  Robins E and Guze SB: Establishment of Diagnostic Validity in Psychiatric Illness: Its Application to Schizophrenia, Am J Psychiatry 1970;126:983-987.
2.  Neuchterlein KH and Dawson ME, A Heuristic Vulnerability/Stress Model of Schizophrenic Episodes, Schizophr Bull (1984) 10 (2): 300-312

# Audit of Clinical Assessment

Assessment is an important aspect of clinical care and involves various aspects that can be audited. The specialist or general practice assessments should provide a person-centred assessment. This ideally should take place in familiar surroundings so that the person and their environment could be better assessed. Communication with the clients should be treated as a partnership and more accessible ways of communicating should be explored. The principles of assessment will be within the context of multi-disciplinary team and in multiprofessional context. The quality of assessment of each client is paramount.

Assessment will be the cornerstone of any health service across all different professionals involved in care. The assessment should be completed in an atmosphere of sympathetic understanding in which the client can feel that professionals have time for him/her and understand his/her difficulties. Also the assessment should focus on and implicitly hold out the possibility of hope and recovery. Without a good quality assessment, meeting the needs of referred clients would prove difficult, and if not completed properly, may prove detrimental to the clients. An assessment by the a health service may include one or more of the following components.

1. Presenting Complaints
2. History of presenting complaints
3. Physical assessment
4. Neurodevelopmental Assessment: A complete neurodevelopmental history will help understand symptoms from a developmental viewpoint.

Psychiatric Assessment (including Mental State Examination)

5. Clinical Psychological Assessment: This assessment will provide detailed psychological formulations on the aetiology and maintenance of mental health problems and help in planning of psychological interventions.
6. Assessment of the child's skills and day to day functioning: Assessing for changes in skills and every day activities will help assessment of impact of the health problem on the clients functioning.
7. Challenging behaviour analysis for learning disabled and very young children: These assessments need to be as detailed as possible and take place in the setting s where the behaviour takes place. Such assessment will look at the antecedents, the behaviours and the consequences of it.
8. Social and Education/Occupational Histories
9. Structured Risk Assessment

Any assessment needs to be summarised as a letter report and a formulation which needs to contain

ICD 10 multi-axial diagnosis
Analysis of need and unmet needs

Recommendations to meet the needs and management proposals.

Assessments need to be co-ordinated by a Key health professional with delegated responsibility of planning and coordinating care. In most situations it is the General practitioner.

Auditing case notes is a frequent and important audit in establishing compliance of basic medical record keeping. Ideally it needs to be performed in a medical setting once every 6 months so that trainees get a good feel of the standards required. In departments where such a turnover of staff is not expected once a year can be sufficient.

## Sampling

Sampling techniques are an important tool in clinical audit. It is important to understand sampling techniques in order to identify and use the correct method. In view of the volume of patients seen it is not physically possible to include all of them in a clinical audit. A sample is a specific collection of the people selected preferable randomly from a population of interest. It however needs to be representative of the entire population.

## Representative or random sampling techniques

In order to get a representative sample of a population, we need to draw the sample in a systematic way so that each and every individual in a sample has an equal opportunity to be selected. There are a number of sampling techniques which are described

Random sampling techniques ensure that selection bias is not introduced regarding who is included in the audit. Four common random sampling techniques are often used in clinical audit

Table 1

1. Simple random sampling: each item in a population has an equal chance of inclusion in the sample. it is simple and easy small populations are involved but difficult to use for large populations
2. Systematic sampling: individuals included in the sample are selected according to an interval between individuals on the population list. For example every 10th person on the list. The interval remains fixed for the entire sample. This method is used often for large populations.
3. Stratified sampling: when samples are required from different groups based on age, gender, diagnosis, ethnic group or geographical area samples can be selected from each of these groups
4. Cluster sampling.: It is sometimes expensive to spread a sample across a big population. A number of clusters are selected at random to represent the population and all people in the selected clusters are included.

Auditing clinical file notes for initial assessments

1. There is a single file including all the notes.
2. All notes are arranged in the required standard
   a. Demography: Administrative staff have entered Full Name and details of the patient, there are addressographs
   b. Referrer's details including date of referral
   c. Contact details including Address and phone number

    d.  Details of General Practitioner

    e.  Details of other agencies involved.

3.  Legal and confidentiality issues
    a.  Consent forms signed by patient/Parent in case of minor
    b.  Consent form signed by clinician
    c.  Concerns about child protection
    d.  Mental capacity Act
    e.  Mental Health Act

4.  People attending the assessment
5.  Presenting difficulties:
6.  History of Presenting Difficulties
7.  Past Medical/ Surgical/ Psychiatric History
8.  Family History
9.  Developmental History
10. Personal History
11. Substance misuse
12. Forensic History
13. Physical examination/ Observation
14. Mental State Examination
15. Cognitive examination
16. Insight
17. Formulation/ Summary
18. Management/ Plan of action/ advice:
19. Therapist signature
20. Clients signature
21. Clinical outcome of severity scores
22. Risk Assessment

## Auditing follow up assessments

1.  Every page has fully completed name, Date of Birth and address
2.  Every entry is dated
3.  Every entry is signed with clinician name printed with Professional designation
4.  Hand writing legible
5.  All entries in black ink
6.  Details of people present at appointment:

7. If there are any corrections they are deleted with a single line and signed and dated with black ink.
8. Letter dictated to General practitioner
9. Letter sent to General practitioner within 2 weeks

## An Example of Audit of medical records

Objectives: To evaluate medical record documentation

Standards:

1. Local trust guideline
2. CNST (Clinical Negligence Scheme for Trusts)
3. Guidelines for Record Keeping (Nursing and Midwifery Council)

Method: Retrospective case note audit. Case notes of patients selected by simple random sampling and filling the predesigned questionnaire

Sample: sample of 30 clients notes

Data analysis: included

1. Documentation of standard details of clients in each case notes
2. Documentation of diagnosis and management plan
3. Evaluation of medication documentation
3. Documentation of subsequent details
4. Documentation of additional entries

*Results analysis*

1. Name, Date of Birth and Address on every page entered in 90% of the notes.
2. All the entries are not dated in 7% case notes
3. Time of assessment not documented in any casenotes
4. All case notes had a signature of clinician. Designation of clinician is not mentioned in 18% notes and in 6% notes it was partly mentioned
5. Referral documentation: available in 100%

6. Diagnosis: In 18% case notes diagnosis was not mentioned
7. Medication: Current mediaction were mentioned in 90%. Rest not on medication.
8. Deletions: It was observed in 9 notes with single stroke deletions.
9. Correspondence: All files had letters to General practitioner within last 6 months.
10. Type of ink used: In 3 cases blue ink used.

*Recommendations*

1. Clinicians should ensure that clients name should be written in all pages
2. Every entry should be signed dated and timed appropriately
3. Signature of the clinician and designation to be entered after each entry with date and time
4. Documentation of source of referrals and acknowledgement should be improved
5. Diagnosis should be mentioned in all the notes in the initial assessment sheet once established
6. Medication and any change of medication and script documentation needs further improvement
7. Any additions should be signed and dated.
8. Deletions should be with only single lines and signed by the clinicians

*Limitations*

1. Small number of notes
2. Difficulty in gathering previous notes
3.

## Auditing what makes a good referral In Child Mental Health Services

Specialist Child and Adolescent Mental Health Services usually function as secondary care teams based within communities at Various localities and take referrals from primary care services which predominantly are general practitioners. The secondary teams work with mental illnesses having high complexity and severity, whereas. The primary care team aims to intervene earlier with the subclinical, milder to moderate cases.

In order to deliver appropriate service to meet individual patients needs it is important for primary care services to make a judgement about whether they can provide the most appropriate help for the family, or if it is essential for a referral to be made to other services. The structure and process needs standardising and is a process that can be audited. The criteria for audit are considered individually but need not be exhaustive.

1. There are standards set by the government recognising need for referrals as a means of providing appropriate care.(1) If they are unclear the referral will be returned to the referrer for further information.
2. It is important that the referrer has met with the child along with parents or carers before child is referred.
3. It is essential that the referral to secondary child health service has been discussed with the parent or carers and the referred child/children and that they are in agreement with the referral being made.
4. If the young person is above 16 years old consent from them without carers consent can be considered.
5. Basic Information to be included in the referral
   - Name and date of birth of referred child
   - Address and telephone number
   - Who has parental responsibility—Parent, carer or social services
   - Surnames if different to child's
   - Details of General Practtioner

6. Reason for Referral
   - What are the main or specific difficulties that need to be addressed.
   - How long has the problem persisted and why is the family seeking help now?
   - Is the context of the problem situation-specific or more generalised?
   - Referrer's understanding of the problems and psychosocial issues involved

7. Other helpful information
   - Who else is living at home and details of relationships between parents if appropriate
   - Name of school, year and any concerns in school
   - Who else has been involved as a professional from health, education or social services and in what capacity?
   - Any previous contact with specialist services. what was the outcome?
   - Has there been any contact with Social Services and what was the outcome?
   - Any known protective or resilience factors
   - Any relevant history i.e. family, life events and/or developmental factors

## Auditing Assessment of Mental Capacity Act

The Mental Capacity Act 2005 for England and Wales(6) sets clear guidance on the definition, assessment and process of addressing any concerns about Mental Capacity. During the assessment process it is very important to assess mental capacity in all cases where appropriate. The criteria for audit are summarized for routine clinical use and can be modified depending on the situation and priorities.

1. Applies to people aged 16 or over
2. Able to make decisions

| A person is unable to make a decision for himself if he is unable |
| --- |
| (a) to understand all the relevant information related to the decision, <br> (b) to retain the information, <br> (c) to weigh that information including the advantages and disadvantages as part of the process of making the decision <br> (d) to communicate his decision. It need not always be in writing or verbal (Any way of objectively identifiable communication—verbal, sign language or any other means). |

3. The decision about mental capacity is made on the basis of a specific situation and at a particular time.

4. Any further decisions of mental capacity need a reassessment.
5. Any act done or decision made under the act for or on behalf of a person who lacks capacity is in that person's best interests
6. Option is given for a person to put his/her wishes and feelings into a written statement if they wish to do so.
7. Carers and relatives and other people involved in caring for the person lacking capacity have been consulted concerning a person's best interests before a decision has been made.
8. Any acts of restraint is justified on the basis of person using it reasonably believing it is necessary to prevent harm to the person who lacks capacity, and restraint used is a proportionate response to the likelihood and seriousness of the harm to others or self.
9. It has been checked that the person has had a Lasting Power of Attorney.
10. Independent Mental Capacity Advocate has been considered to support a person who lacks capacity but has no one to speak for them.
11. The person has/has not made a decision in advance to refuse treatment if they should lack capacity in the future.
12. If an advance decision has been made the decision is in writing, signed and witnessed.
13. Any ill treatment or neglect of a person who lacks capacity is considered a criminal offence and is reported as such. A person found guilty of such an offence may be liable to imprisonment.

## Auditing assessment of deliberate self harm in young people.

Auditing self harm standards is a very useful tool in auditing the multidisciplinary nature of the process and the need for coordination. A typical audit may involve the following steps.

Introduction

Deliberate self-harm (DSH) is common in adolescents in many countries of the world. The prevalence increases from the age of 12 years and especially so in girls. Most common form of self-harm is by self-poisoning. During the final six years of a study period, Hawton et al (1996)(3) found that paracetamol was involved in 54.7% of overdoses, compared with

19.5% in 1976-1981. A minority of persons had previous psychiatric treatment. Most frequently, the problems that they said they had were in relationships with parents, followed by difficulties with friends, school and social isolation. The majority of young people who reported previous DSH said that the events had not come to medical attention. Nearly 10% (9.4%) had harmed themselves again within year of an episode and 19.3% had done so during the five years of the study. There was some indication that repetition was most common in young people who were discharged from emergency departments without a full psychosocial assessment.

There is evidence that DSH occurs far more frequently in the population than is reflected in general hospital figures. A cross sectional survey (4) using an anonymous self report questionnaire of DSH of 6,020 pupils aged 15 and 16 years who attended in 41 schools in England showed that 398 (6.9%) of them had deliberately harmed themselves in the previous. Only 12.6% of these events had resulted in the young person going to hospital.

The NICE guidelines makes evidence based guidance for the physical, psychological and social assessment and treatment of people in primary and secondary care in the first 48 hours after having self-harmed. For the purpose of this guideline, the term self-harm is defined as 'self-poisoning or injury, irrespective of the apparent purpose of the act'. It recognises that self-harm is an expression of personal distress, not an illness, and there are many varied reasons for a person to harm him or herself.

The guideline is relevant to all people aged 8 years of age and older who have self-harmed. Where it refers to children and young people, this applies to all people who are between 8 and 16 years of age inclusive. However, local services vary the upper age limit depending upon whether a young person is in full-time education or not.

Some generic recommendations are for all people who self harm. The role of primary services in most circumstances of self-poisoning should be to urgently refer to the nearest emergency department, because the nature and quantity of the ingested substances may not be clearly known to the person who has self-poisoned, making accurate risk assessment difficult. The emergency department provides the main services for people who self-harm. All people who have self-harmed should be offered a preliminary psychosocial assessment at triage following an act of self-harm.

A psychosocial assessment should not be delayed until after medical treatment is complete, unless life-saving medical treatment is needed, or the patient is unconscious or otherwise incapable of being assessed.

Children and young people who self-harm have a number of special needs, given their vulnerability. All children or young people who have self-harmed should normally be admitted overnight to a paediatric ward and assessed fully the following day before discharge. A paediatrician should normally have overall responsibility for the treatment and care of children and young people who have been admitted following an act of self-harm. During admission to a paediatric ward following self-harm, the Child and Adolescent Mental Health Team should undertake assessment and provide consultation for the young person, his or her family, the paediatric team and social services and education staff as appropriate.

All cases of self-harm need to be taken seriously as there is an increased risk of eventual death by suicide, but the evidence base for effective intervention is sparse (4). Ideally all under-18s who have deliberately harmed themselves should be seen and systematically assessed by Emergency services. Child mental health professionals play a consulting role. All assessments need to be completed before discharge, as otherwise follow-up contact is difficult. There are many instruments for assessing suicide risk in young people, none perfect, but they can be very useful for multi-disciplinary teams in promoting standardised and comprehensive emergency assessments. The major triage decisions are whether the young person can go home safely, whether his or her care needs to be taken over temporarily by social services and whether he or she should be admitted to psychiatric care. Overnight admission is recommended, ideally to a paediatric ward or, for 14–to 16-year-olds, to a ward for adolescents, but this is not always possible. Misuse of drugs and alcohol merits special inquiry and attention, as does the possibility of abuse.

The suicide rate for 15-to 19-year-old males, especially by hanging, increased markedly from 1970 to 1998 (5). Comorbidity is common and underlines the need for full evaluations, both of the child or adolescent and of the family and social circumstances.

Problem: There are wide variations in the assessment and care pathways used locally for children and young people who have deliberately harmed themselves. The professional practitioners who work in healthcare services work in different ways in different organisations. Much of this variation remains despite clear guidelines from the National Institute for Health and Clinical Excellence (NICE) (2) and it may affect the quality of care delivered.

Setting: A acute hospital in an urban district with an Accident and Emergency department. There are care pathways used by the service specifically for self harm starting from the time of their attendance in the emergency department through their transition to paediatric service and the child and adolescent mental health service to discharge and follow-up.

Design: A proforma design that is a summary of key recommendations in the NICE guidelines for assessing children and adolescents who present to hospital emergency departments after they have harmed themselves is essential. Scrutinising the clinical assessment notes for patients who meet the criteria over a accepted period of time so as to get a statistically significant number of clients is essential. Strategies for change: Audit of local standards carried out against the benchmark of the standards that presented as acceptable by NICE is essential. In particular, understanding if the process used by the hospital is evidence-informed and the various hospital departments are all aligned to achieve a common goal can be assessed efficiently. Consequently, such audits examine the concurrence and disparities between the NICE recommendations and clinical practice as children and young people pass through in a district general hospital and back into the community-based services.

Results: can be presented as numbers or percentage. Percentages make comparisions of reaudit easier.

Various possible Conclusions include:

The staff who are involved with children and young people who harm themselves should receive more training about the process of self-harm and assessment of, mainly, young people who are involved.

1.   The different roles and responsibilities of the staff and departments that are involved (routinely they are the emergency department, the paediatric service and Specialist CAMHS) should be clear.

2.  There must be good information sharing between the hospital departments and services involved if there is to be an effective, coherent and seamless care pathway that provides for effective and smooth transitions for patients between departments and clear for the clinicians and managers and patients.

3.  Good leadership and a quality improvement plan is required, which is based on good local evidence and a community-wide approach, in order to improve the quality of the processes of care sufficiently to reduce the potential for young people to fail to receive adequate assessment of and intervention with their psychosocial problems. The NICE guidelines, that were prepared in collaboration with all the relevant specialties, are available to assist professional and general mangers to standardise care pathways locally and develop local practice.

## Discussion

This study design and a small sample size should allow clinical data to be gathered in a standardized, comprehensive and efficient way. Retrospective case note studies are dependent on the diligence with which the original clinical information is collected and recorded. Occasionally, information obtained may not be recorded. Illegible handwriting or the use of undecipherable acronyms can make it difficult to interpret the information. Such ambiguous information cannot be audited accurately. Unfortunately, it is also not possible to confirm whether all details of management had been recorded, particularly referral to mental health services from Accident and Emergency. However the more common referrals from Paediatric wards for Child psychiatrist assessments are formal referral requests and are usually available for audit.

The use of a proforma for recording data overcomes some of the problems that may arise in a non-standardized collection of data. Using all consecutive young people up to their 17th birthday who presented with deliberate self-harm can solve some of the sampling biases and can represent a random sample. The over inclusive nature of NICE guideline definition of self harm seems to be under recognised by many assessment teams especially with regard to accidental ingestion, superficial cutting and substance misuse and intoxication.

A concise protocol, which highlights these aspects, would not only ensure that crucial information is not missed, but also serve to raise concerns and encourage referral for specialist input. According to NICE guidelines all children presenting to accident and emergency with deliberate self harm need to be admitted and a detailed psychosocial assessment carried out.

Although it is desirable for children to be admitted to a paediatric ward, some older adolescents are often admitted to an adult medical ward. This is more likely to occur if they are initially assessed in the adult accident and emergency. Initial presentation to the adult accident and emergency would also explain the small number referred to Child psychiatry and assessed by the Adult Mental Health Service, even though they are within the remit of child psychiatry.

It would be useful to consider the possible reasons, and identify solutions, for the results of such audits. Resources may be a factor. Authorities with responsibility for commissioning health service provision should identify the resources required and work with provider health services to ensure that appropriate and relevant arrangements are in place for the management of young people who self-harm. Another possible likely factor may be the lack of appropriate training for junior medical and nursing staff in accident and emergency in management of deliberate self-harm in young people. Evidence for this can be a lack of psychosocial assessments recorded in the notes. Appropriate training sessions can be organized on a regular basis for each intake of junior staff, within the constraints of the demands placed on them by other specialist services.

Finally, young people presenting with self-harm may not be referred to CAMHS by accident and emergency staff if the local specialist service is perceived to be unresponsive. This could be addressed by a collaborative approach to training staff in accident and emergency complimented by a dedicated DSH team that can respond, without delay, to requests for psychiatric assessment. Overnight admission to a suitable ward usually ensures assessment the next day under current policy and also prevent the process from occurring in an inappropriate environment such as a busy accident and emergency.

Guidelines are most useful when they are influential enough to change practice. The NICE guidelines with respect to the management of deliberate self-harm in young people, appear to suffer from the drawback of not having the endorsement of other specialities such as Paediatrics and Accident and Emergency Medicine especially with regard to psychosocial assessments. Guidelines produced locally in consultation with these specialities are likely to be more influential and have the required impact on services.

The Royal college of psychiatrists has embarked on a ambitious proactive audit which requires the provision of additional resources. Audits can demonstrate that the guidelines are not being implemented in a district hospital. There may be similar difficulties nationally, as summarized above, possibly due to lack of endorsement, not only by other professional bodies, but also by psychiatrists. This may be due to perceived inability to apply the guidelines within current resources and prompts an ethical question about whether alternative avenues should be explored or whether the Royal College of Psychiatrists should advocate strongly for the provision of sufficient paediatric in-patient resources to effect these guidelines. The guidelines, and the evidence on which they are based, may need to be reviewed. Meanwhile, we believe that best practice as defined by these guidelines should not be compromised due to lack of resources.

1.  *http://www.every-child-matters.org.uk/Home*
2.  National Institute of clinical excellance(2004). Self-harm: The short-term physical and psychological management and secondary prevention of self-harm in primary and secondary care, NICE guidelines, July 2004.
3.  The British Journal of Psychiatry 169: 202-208 (1996) Deliberate self-poisoning and self-injury in children and adolescents under 16 years of age in Oxford, 1976-1993
4.  K Hawton, J Fagg and S Simkin: University Department of Psychiatry, Warneford Hospital, Oxford. BMJ 2002;325:1207-1211 ( 23 November )
5.  McClure, G. M. G. (2001) Suicide in children and adolescents in England and Wales 1970-1998. British Journal of Psychiatry, 178, 469-474.
6.  The Mental Capacity Act 2005 for England and Wales, Department of Health, united Kingdom

# Survey and Audit

Surveys serve various functions. The most common one is similar to the the audit in terms of evaluating some basic assumptions that we all make in routine clinical practice. In research it is a powerful preliminary step in making decisions about priorities for further research.

But a survey is different from an audit and the difference is exemplified in this chapter with examples.

## Survey of Eating Disorder Services

The National Institute for Clinical Excellence (NICE) in the United Kingdom has published clinical guidelines for management of Eating disorders. These include standards for specific core interventions in the treatment and management of anorexia nervosa, bulimia nervosa and related eating disorders. In order to determine what services were already being provided within a particular service a survey would serve as a basic tool. It can be used as a baseline to evaluate standards of care being delivered in the form of an audit.and to identify the main areas requiring service development.

Aims / Objectives

The aims of the survey are to ascertain the different practices within health services with regard to the treatment and management of eating disorders and to identify areas of good practice and those requiring further augmentation. The survey would also provide a baseline from which to work when planning future service developments. It is exploratory and needs no comparision standards.

The aims of an audit would be to have a set of pre agreed standards that any standard service needs to offer and compare current practices to the gold standard.

## Methodology

In terms of methodology both a survey and audit need a questionnaire based on the criteria outlined in the NICE Guidance. The sample population could be based in the community services or in the inpatient services. The process of sampling depends on the sample size rather than weather it is an audit or survey. However financial funding in research allows for greater numbers to be included in surveys.

A research survey needs to be evaluated by a ethics committee to validate the research methodology and patient safety. It needs to meet the requirements of the Research Governance Framework. An audit does not usually require such review and approval. However the clinical and managerial leads have a duty to ensure that the audit is a clinical practice improvement exercise within a preagreed priority with a need for evaluation of quality and if a problem is identified they are required to proactively address it within the context of clinical governance.

The research Governance Framework provides a set of Standards that all researchers should achieve. Their purpose is to: Table 1

–Ensure the dignity, rights, safety and well being of the public

–Improve the quality of research being carried out

–Prevent poor performance and adverse events

–Prevent misconduct and fraud

Table 2: Research Governance Standards
The Research Governance Framework is split into five domains, which are:

| |
|---|
| –Ethics |
| –Science |
| –Information |
| –Health and Safety and Employment |
| –Finance and Intellectual property |

## Planning a questionnaire for Survey and Audit

1. Physical and Mental Health Assessment of people with eating disorders should be comprehensive and include physical, psychological and social needs, and a comprehensive assessment of risk to self

Do you have a standard assessment?

1. Mental health standard assessment—Refer to audit on assessment
2. physical health assessment

What physical assessment / investigations to undertake?

Height and weight
Blood tests
BP and pulse
General Physical examination
Systemic Physical Examination
Bone scan
Ovarian scan
ECG

2. When the patient is in the community management is shared between primary and secondary care. There should be clear agreement among each healthcare professional about the responsibility for monitoring patients with eating disorders

Is there clear agreement and liaison?

Yes
No

Is there a protocol in place?

Yes
No

3. Clients with eating disorders wanting help need to be assessed and managed without delay

How quickly do you assess patients who are referred?

Within 1 week
Within 2-4 weeks
Later than 4 weeks/ 1 month

How quickly does treatment begin?

Immediately
In 1 week
In 3-4 weeks
After 4 weeks/ a month
Wait and watch

Which professional groups are involved in the treatment?

Psychiatrist
Nurse Therapist / CPN
Family Therapist
Psychologist
Paediatrician
Dietitian
CPN
Social Work Therapist
General Physician
Physician
Psychotherapist
CIT Team
Specialist Unit

4. Family members should be included in treatment of clients with eating disorders

Are you able to offer family interventions?

Yes
No

How quickly are families seen?
Immediately
In 1 week
In 3-4 weeks
After 4 weeks/ a month

5. Patients and carers should be provided with education and information on the nature, course and treatment of eating disorders

Do you provide information and education to patients and carers?

Standardised information given
Adhoc information given

Written information given
Verbal information given

6. In young people with eating disorders, growth and development should be closely monitored.

Yes
No

7. Where development is delayed or growth is stunted despite adequate nutrition, paediatric advice should be sought.

Yes
No

8. Refer young patients with diagnosed eating disorders by a paediatrician
   Yes

Yes
No

9. Do you monitor growth as well as weight and chart it?

Yes
No

10. adults with eating disorders are referred to a physician for physical evaluation

Yes
No

11. Healthcare professionals assessing young people with eating disorders should be alert to indicators of abuse and should remain so throughout treatment

Have all professionals seeing children with eating disorders have training in child protection—Yes/No

Are there standardised forms to assess for child protection issues—Yes/No

Is the team team sufficiently aware of the child protection issues specifically in young people with eating disorders—Yes/No

12. The right to confidentiality of clients with eating disorders should be respected

Is there a confidentiality policy—Yes/No

Are all team members aware of confidentiality policy—Yes/No

Is confidentiality assessed routinely—Yes/No

## Treatment of bulimia nervosa

Steps 1-12 apply followed by

13. Patients with bulimia nervosa should be encouraged to follow a self-help programme initially

Do you offer a self help programme—Yes/No

Self help programme is standardised—Yes/No

14. Adolescents with bulimia nervosa may be treated with Cognitive behaviour Therapy–Yes/No

Cognitive behaviour Therapy is adapted as needed to suit their age, circumstances and level of development, and including the family as appropriate–Yes/No

15. The great majority of patients with bulimia nervosa are preferably treated in an outpatient setting–Yes/No

16. Psychiatric admission for people with bulimia nervosa if occasionally required should normally be undertaken in a setting with experience of managing this disorder–Yes/No

17. Therapeutic options available for eating disorders

Dietetics
Adequate physical assessment and monitoring
Admission to in-patient setting
Family Therapy
Psychotherapy
Occupational Therapy
Psychologist
Community support
CBT
Individual Therapy
Behavioural Therapy / Advice
Day Unit
Assessment
Group Therapy
Medication for co-morbid disorders
Physical monitoring

18. Do you give patients a choice?–Yes/No

19. Does your team feel that it has the required competencies to offer this treatment?

Yes
No

20. Do you liaise with the school or other appropriate agencies in all cases?–Yes/No

21. Do you inform patients and carers about physical risk?–Yes/No

22. When making the decision to feed a person against their will, the legal basis for any such action must be clear–Yes/No

The above questionnaire would meet all the standards for a survey. For this to be converted into a audit all the yes/no questions need to be compared against a essential gold standard. For severe illnesses with adverse outcomes like eating disorders such a gold standard is more likely to be 100%. In less risky areas a compliance of 80% would constitute an acceptable result. However these need to be agreed before hand before the standards in use are measured and compared again acceptable standards.

A Survey Questionnaire about client or carers assessment of experience

Name (optional): diagnosis?
For each question, please circle or tick the answer that is closest to what you think.

*Before the assessment*

1. How well were you informed about the assessment before you attended the first appointment?

| ☐ | ☐ | ☐ | ☐ | ☐ |
|---|---|---|---|---|
| Bad | poor | Satisfactory | Good | Very Good |

2. Was the information you were given before assessment adequate

| ☐ | ☐ | ☐ | ☐ | ☐ |
|---|---|---|---|---|
| Bad | poor | Satisfactory | Good | Very Good |

Did you get details about                                        ☑
i)–name and profession of person seeing the child            ☐
ii)–questions that you would be asked                         ☐

iii)–how long it would take to make a diagnosis ☐
iv)–all the different parts of the assessment process ☐
    What other information would you have liked

..........................................................................................................
..........................................................................................................

## *Assessment*

3.  Did you like the professionals who saw you

☐              ☐              ☐              ☐              ☐
_____
Bad          poor         Satisfactory        Good         Very Good

4.  Were you/Was your child happy to attend the assessment?

_____

5.

☐              ☐              ☐              ☐              ☐
_____
Bad          poor         Satisfactory        Good         Very Good

What might have made a difference

..........................................................................................................
..........................................................................................................
..........................................................................................................

6.  Did you feel that the professional(s) listened to you?

☐              ☐              ☐              ☐              ☐
_____
Bad          poor         Satisfactory        Good         Very Good

7.  Was it easy to talk in the assessment?

☐              ☐              ☐              ☐              ☐
_____
Bad          poor         Satisfactory        Good         Very Good

8.  How were you treated by the people who saw you?

☐              ☐              ☐              ☐              ☐
_____
Bad          poor         Satisfactory        Good         Very Good

9. Was there given enough time to discuss your concerns?

☐         ☐              ☐              ☐              ☐

Bad        poor         Satisfactory      Good         Very Good

*After the assessment*

10. How was the outcome of the assessment communicated to you?

☐         ☐              ☐              ☐              ☐

Bad        poor         Satisfactory      Good         Very Good

11. Do you have any suggestions?

........................................................................................................
........................................................................................................
........................................................................................................

12. At the end of the assessment, were you given extra information regarding your problems and treatment?

Verbal                                                    ☐
Written                                                   ☐
Information booklet.                                       ☐
Self-help leaflets                                        ☐
Voluntary agencies                                        ☐
Information about other services                          ☐
Any other                                                 ☐
(please specify) ...............................................................
Any other please specify...............................................

13. Overall, how satisfied were you with the assessment process?

☐         ☐              ☐              ☐              ☐

Bad        poor         Satisfactory      Good         Very Good

# Fluoxetine Survey

Fluoxetine is a commonly used antidepressant and a survey to identify common side effects can be easily planned. A sample example is given.

*Identified Risks Experienced*

- Increased anxiety in the initial period                    Agree/Disagree
- Any allergies to a particular drug                          Agree/Disagree
- Increase of suicidal thoughts (if any apparent initially)   Agree/Disagree
- Interactions with other medications                        Agree/Disagree
- Parents to control medication                              Agree/Disagree

*Probable side effects*

- Headaches                    Agree/Disagree
- Dizziness                    Agree/Disagree
- Nausea and Vomiting          Agree/Disagree
- Diarrhoea                    Agree/Disagree
- Sleeplessness                Agree/Disagree
- Weight loss                  Agree/Disagree
- Skin reactions               Agree/Disagree
- Sexual dysfunction (rarely)  Agree/Disagree

*Sudden withdrawal symptoms*

- Tummy upset         Agree/Disagree
- Flu like symptoms   Agree/Disagree
- Sleep disturbances  Agree/Disagree
- Sweating            Agree/Disagree

# Management and Treatment audits

Following the assessment, the need for treatment/interventions from the health service or from other services will usually be identified. The health service has a duty of care to use interventions that will be evidence based in 'what works' for specific people with specific identified health problems. There is a need to justify evidence supporting the use of psychological, pharmacological and other more specific interventions. Sometimes however there may be a need to extrapolate evidence based interventions. For example using medications effective in adults in a population of children and adolescents or in vulnerable groups of people like old age or people with learning disabilities. In such situations all uncertainities need to be discussed among peers and communicated to patients clearly and should be used after consent.

Treatment options and interventions that will be offered will usually depend on the therapeutic skills available within the local team or area. However the local team needs to be aware of national guidelines based evidence and should have the resources and training to deliver those services that are considered essential within an effective evidence based supportive therapeutic environment with individualised care plans. Multidisciplinary team members and professionals will bring skills to the team. The teams should additionally be committed to continued professional development in regards to the use of different therapeutic modalities recommended as acceptable evidence based treatments.

Some overriding principles of management need to be kept in mind

1. Evidence based treatment and management strategies should be used wherever such evidence is available.
2. In line with Child Care legislation, the young person, their wishes and needs remain paramount in any intervention package developed. In such situations interventions will be aimed at the specific needs of the young person "a child centred approach". If the young person is unable to make a decision with regard to the best intervention or the one they prefer the treatment will be discussed with their relatives and professionals involved in their case, then a decision should be taken in the young person's best interest.
3. The family and individual are key in the successful implementation of the treatment decisions and plans. Therefore they need to be involved and their consent and opinions sought and in agreement with the care plans.
4. Intervention strategies will have to involve multi agency co-operation and involvement where required with a nominated care coordinator.
5. It will be impossible and undesirable for the service to try and offer every intervention the patient may need. These need to be addressed through Multi-agency co-operation.
6. An important point to acknowledge is that other professionals and agencies can deliver better services in certain circumstances, for example, educational interventions by qualified teaching staff. Such services in primary care need to be involved even if they are being managed in specialist care.

## An example proforma for auditing Prescriptions

### Prescription Writing Audit Standards

#### General Requirements for all Prescriptions

Prescriptions form an important part of the medical management process and requires strategies and procedures in place to avoid potentially harmful errors. The prescriptions should be based on national guidelines and legislation, and apply to all prescriptions including in-patient charts, outpatient and prescriptions issued in outpatient clinics.

- All prescriptions must be written:
    1. Clearly
    2. Legibly
    3. With indelible ink

- Patient Identification & Details must be clear and must be checked
    1. The patient's full name, address, date of birth and hospital number must appear on all prescriptions. In hospital inpatient settings these should be checked with the wrist band or with the patient to confirm identity before dispensing drugs.
    2. Age, height and weight must be stated on all paediatric prescriptions (under 16 years).

- Drug Name
    1. The international approved drug name must be written in block letters with frequency and times of day when it is to be taken.
    2. Do not use chemical descriptions or abbreviations for drug names. They increase the risk of medication errors
    3. The bioavailablity of some medications may vary between different brands, and these should be prescribed by brand name, such drugs include:

| |
|---|
| Aminophylline modified release |
| Ciclosporin |
| Lithium |
| Theophylline modified release |

It may sometimes be appropriate or necessary to use the brand name, in addition to the approved name, for other medicines to avoid confusion. These need to be in the hospital prescription protocol and need to be discussed with the pharmacist.

- Formulation, dose and administration
    If different formulations or multiple dose strengths of a single medication preparation are available, it is important that details of formulation and dose are correctly written on the prescription.

It is also important to state the way or through a device through which medication is administered to ensure the patient receives the correct medication.

- Drug Dose
    1. The dose of medication and route of administration and frequency must be written on all prescriptions. Please avoid use of decimal points. It is preferable to write it as whole numbers with appropriate metric measure following it. If decimal points are unavoidable, a zero must be put in front of the decimal point where there is no other figure. Example 0.5mg.
    2. Except milligrams (mg) all other measures like micrograms, nanograms and other units must be written in full and not abbreviated
    3. In some cases gm (grams), ml (millilitres), and mg (milligrams) are acceptable abbreviations but not generally recommended.
    4. The concentration of liquid preparations should be stated in all cases.

- Route of administration
    Route of administration should be specified in all cases. When prescribing by different routes doses may not be equivalent in which case available evidence need to be used for working out equivalent doses. If there is a difference separate prescriptions for each route of administration must be written.

There are some acceptable abbreviations are:

| | |
|---|---|
| IV intra-venous | IM intra-muscular |
| SC sub-cutaneous | PO / O oral |
| NG naso-gastric | PEG via peg tube |
| JEJ via jejunostomy tube | S/L sub-lingual |
| PR rectal | PV vaginal |
| Top topical | INH inhaled |
| NEB nebulised | |
| LE left eye | |

- Frequency
    The dose frequency must be stated on all prescriptions.

Some medications can be prescribed as "as required" medications. In such cases the maximum allowed dose and a minimum dose interval must be specified. It is considered as good practice to state the indication for any "as required" medication.

Directions should be in English without abbreviation ideally. However some traditional Latin abbreviations are acceptable:

| | |
|---|---|
| o.d. | daily |
| o.m. or mane | in the morning |
| b.d. | twice daily |
| o.n. or nocte | at night |
| t.d.s. | three times daily |
| stat | immediately |
| q.d.s. | four times daily |
| a.c. | before food |
| p.r.n. | when required |
| p.c. | after food |

when prescribing medications for a limited time like antibiotics this must be stated on the prescription.

- Prescriber's Signature & Date
  All prescriptions must be signed and dated by the prescriber and contact details written.

## Prescribing In-patient Medication Charts

*Inpatient medication charts need additional standards.*

A new chart must be written for each admission, and the old chart must be discontinued (by crossing and cancelling through the front page) when the patient is discharged.

Charts that are no longer in use must be crossed through on the front page, but information on the chart should be visible and should not be obscured.

Patient's name, date of birth and address with hospital number must be stated on each page of the chart to reduce the risk of error.

- All prescriptions should have a Allergy box
    1. This section must be completed compulsorily in all cases after checking old records and with patient. It needs to be signed and dated.
    2. If an allergy is known or documented all available information regarding the type of allergy, should be documented on the chart.
    3. Medication must not be administered if this section is not completed.

- Hospital: Details must be completed and kept up to date whenever any changes are made.
- Ward: Details must be completed and kept up to date whenever any changes are made.
- Consultant: Details must be completed and kept up to date whenever any changes are made.
- Weight / Height / Body surface area
  Weight must be stated on all paediatric charts.
  Weight should be included on adult charts when appropriate for medication dosage.
  Height should also be recorded when body surface area is used to calculate dosage.

- Extra and supplementary medication charts & multiple medication charts

This section should have records of other medication charts in use. As a general rule, drugs prescribed on supplementary charts like drug detoxification and warfarin should also be recorded on the main chart, with a reference to the supplementary chart on the prescription.

If there are multiple medication charts they must be recorded sequentially as 1 of 2, 2 of 2 etc numerically.

- *Prescription of once only medicines*
  Should always be recorded on the chart before it is given

All sections of the prescription must be completed
Record time of administration using 24-hour clock format.

- As required medicines
  Should always be recorded on the chart before it is given
  All sections of the prescription must be completed
  Record time of administration using 24-hour clock format.
  Include indication for as required medicines.

- Prescribing Regular Medications
  Should always be recorded on the chart before it is given
  All sections of the prescription must be completed
  Record time of administration using 24-hour clock format.

Date of prescription starting and on day of administering need to be recorded

Complete the month and year at the top of the chart.

Date the prescription using the original start date and not the date a chart is re-written
Record Route, dose & dose change
Allways follow guidelines for prescribing doses and using abbreviations.
Specify the route of administration.
Record appropriate administration time using 24-hour clock format.
When a dose change is necessary, cancel with a cross through the original dose box and write the date of change, new route and new dose, sign or initial the change.
If there is a need for Special instructions record them clearly

- Discontinuation
  When a medicine is discontinued this must be clearly indicated by cancel marking a Z through the drug name and the end of the treatment. The discontinuation must be signed and dated.

  Drugs with a limited course of treatment like antibiotics should have a bar line marked on the chart to indicate the end of treatment, and when the course is finished the prescription should be crossed through as for regular medications.

- Pharmacist check box
- **A pharmacist's signature indicates that the prescription has been screened for accuracy and appropriateness. The pharmacist should also date the entry.**

If a dose of medication is not administered for any reason, it must be entered on the chart, and an entry made in the patient's medical records.

If the prescriber requires a dose to be omitted, a cross must be entered in the appropriate box.

- Intravenous & sub-cutaneous infusions for administration
  The prescriber must sign the appropriate box to indicate that a infusion is required. If the prescriber does not initial or sign this section, the infusion must not be repeated.

# AN AUDIT OF SEDATIVE PRECRIPTION AMONG ADMITTED PATIENTS

ABSTRACT

AIMS AND METHODS
Patient records from patients admitted to Inpatient Unit were analysed for a period of a week. Sedative medications prescribed was audited to assess the indications compared to indications mentioned in the British National Formulary (1) and World Health Organisation Guidelines. The drugs prescribed including dosage and length of prescription were noted. An intervention of regular presentation and discussion in audit meetings followed by reminders was circulated to clinical staff after each cycle every 6 months.

RESULTS
A significant decrease in sedative use was evident in the initial period but further decrease after a year were not observed.

CLINICAL IMPLICATIONS
Continuous evaluation and feedback by audit can improve the quality of management of insomnia and reduce sedative use among inpatients.

INTRODUCTION

Sleep disturbances are common among patients admitted to inpatient wards. Non pharmacological management of insomnia remains an effective and practical method but medication continues to be a significantly used.

Sedatives are used to treat sleep disturbances in acutely ill patients with disturbed sleep especially if therapeutic medication takes weeks to have an effect. The number of prescriptions of benzodiazepines has been decreasing significantly ever since the CSM warning regarding dependance (Scottish Health Service Advisory Council 1994) (4). The British National Formulary and the World Health Organisation Guide to Mental Health in Primary care, advises restricting use of sedatives to primary insomnia and for periods not more than 3 weeks.

Often, in the interim, additional, 'as required' doses of medication can be used to calm patients in psychiatric wards. 20 to 50% of people on acute psychiatric wards are written up for 'as required' doses of medication. In this situation, a doctor prescribes the frequency and upper limit of dose, and the drug is then given at the discretion of clinical staff. This common current practice has no support from randomised trials. Current practice is based on clinical experience and habit rather than high quality evidence. Current practice, therefore, outside of a well designed, conducted and reported randomised trial, is therefore difficult to justify.(Whicher E 2004). In the treatment of depression, evidence for the efficacy of adding a benzodiazepine to an antidepressant is restricted to short term only and must be balanced judiciously against possible harms including development of dependence and accident proneness, on the one hand, and against continued suffering following no response and drop-out, on the other (2).

The adult inpatient units provide inpatient services for acute adult wards, intensive care, rehabilitation unit and elderly wards. The care provided is varied and suited for audit of prescriptions and case notes. The hospital has a policy of prescribing lormetazepam if required for insomnia. Other medications are only used if it is ineffective or if side effects occur. All units are staffed with nurses.

This study aimed to assess the prescription patterns of sedatives and the non pharmacological measures recorded in the notes for all patients prescribed sedatives and to evaluate the effect of intervention in minimising sedative prescription, encourage non pharmacological interventions.and introduce guidelines for sedative use.

## METHOD

An audit tool was designed to ascertain if each of the standards were met (Table 1). Prescription charts of all patients in all the units were reviewed as a cross sectional survey and all patients who were prescribed sedatives were selected. Prescriptions were only included as sedatives if they were exclusively prescribed for administration at night and belonged to benzodiazepines, antihistaminergics or newer hypnotics. Benzodiazepines prescribed for rapid tranquilisation were excluded. The sedative prescribed, duration of prescription and dosage of medication were recorded. Case notes of patients prescribed sedatives were reviewed for explicit indications, regular management reviews of medication and non pharmacological interventions.

## FOLLOW UP AND INTERVENTION

The audits were repeated at intervals of six months Including all inpatients completing three audit cycles and results were discussed in audit meetings after each cycle involving all members of the multidisciplinary teams. Minutes of audit meetings, and copies of audit with explicit guidelines for sedative prescription was circulated to all health teams including inpatient nursing staff. All new junior doctors at time of induction were informed. Data was analysed without any blinding.

## RESULTS

Sets of notes were analysed at 6 month intervals. The patient groups did not differ in terms of their age and sex. Prescription of sedatives decreased in initial periods but there was significant room for improvement.

## DISCUSSION

There was a reduction in number of prescriptions, duration of prescriptions and change in medications being prescribed. Despite these trends there was a continuation of longer term prescription and continued use of newer sedatives.

The role of the pharmacist in mediating such a change has been unexplored in this audit. The nationally formulated guidelines may help in sustaining lower sedative use among inpatients.

Audit and feedback continues to be widely used as a strategy to improve professional practice. It appears logical that healthcare professionals would be prompted to modify their practice if given feedback that their clinical practice was inconsistent with that of their peers or accepted guidelines. Yet, audit and feedback has not been found to be consistently effective. Audit and feedback can be effective in improving professional practice. When it is effective, the effects are generally small to moderate. The absolute effects of audit and feedback are more likely to be larger when baseline adherence to recommended practice is low (Jamtvedt G). The lack of nationally formulated guidelines on use of sedatives and absence of local trust policies on differentiating use of hypnotics for tranquilisation and sedation may blur the distinction. This needs further investigation by assessment of attitudes of clinical team members.

Limitations This audit assessed only the documentation of all prescription charts and case notes of patients prescribed sedatives. The clinical assessment and review may have included non pharmacological management and review of sedative medication and may not have been communicated verbally than by writing. Weak intervention strategies, small sample size, differences between community teams and inpatient units could have accounted for these findings. The prescriptions were from eight psychiatric teams and though consultants were the same throughout the period of the audit, junior doctors tended to change every 6 months. Despite these limitations a positive change suggests the audit as a good measure indicating need for change and monitoring progress. The intervention strategies needs to be refined, focussed and more intensive to effect more significant changes.

## Table 1
Criteria assessed for all patients

| | percentage required to meet standards(n) |
|---|---|
| number of patients | 100% |
| hypnotic used as | |
|     as required | 0 |
|     regular | 0 |
| | |
| within bnf dose | 100% |
| hypnotic started | |
|     before admission | |
|     after admission | |
|     unknown | 0% |
| | |
| duration used | |
|     less than 3 weeks | 100% |
|     3 weeks to 3 months | 0% |
|     more than 3 months | 0% |
| clinical indication | |
|     transient insomnia | 0 |
|     short term insomia | 0 |
|     others | 0 |
| | |
| lormetazepam used if medication indication indicated | 100% |
| | |
| other sedative used only if lormetazepam ineffective | 0% |
| | |
| duration prescribed not more than one week | 100% |
| | |
| hypnotic administered before 1am | 0% |
| sleep hygiene/diary | 100% |

*Dr. PS Reddy*

## Table 2

| | | | | |
|---|---|---|---|---|
| Total number | 62 | 68 | 67 | 66 |
| | | | | |
| Hypnotic use | 19 | 22 | 12 | 13 |
| As required | 18 | 20 | 9 | 11 |
| Regular | 1 | 2 | 3 | 2 |
| | | | | |
| Within BNF Dose | 19 | 21 | 12 | 13 |
| Started | | | | |
| Before admission | 0 | 4 | 0 | 3 |
| After admission | 19 | 13 | 12 | 10 |
| Unknown | 0 | 1 | 0 | 0 |
| | | | | |
| Duration used | | | | |
| Less than 3 weeks | 12 | 3 | 7 | 10 |
| 3 weeks to 3 months | 5 | 7 | 5 | 3 |
| More than 3 months | 2 | 7 | 0 | 0 |
| | | | | |
| Clinical indication | | | | |
| Transient insomnia | 1 | 1 | 6 | 0 |
| Short term insomnia | 0 | 0 | 2 | 11 |
| Others | 18 | 16 | 4 | 2 |
| | | | | |
| Duration prescribed | | | | |
| 1 week | 1 | 0 | 2 | 1 |
| 2 weeks | 4 | 1 | 4 | 0 |
| 3 weeks | 0 | 0 | 1 | 1 |
| 4 weeks | 6 | 20 | 4 | 9 |
| 6 weeks | 1 | 0 | 0 | 1 |
| 8 weeks | 0 | 0 | 8 | 1 |
| 14 weeks | 7 | 0 | 0 | 0 |
| Unclear | 0 | 1 | 0 | 0 |

| | | | | |
|---|---|---|---|---|
| Lormetazepam used | 16 | 10 | 4 | 8 |
| Other sedative used | 3 | 12 | 8 | 5 |
| Hypnotic before 1 PM | 14 | 20 | 10 | 8 |
| Sleep hygiene/ diary | 0 | 0 | 0 | 0 |

# REFERENCES

1. Joint Formulary Committee. British National Formulary. [edition number] ed. London: British Medical Association and Royal Pharmaceutical Society of Great Britain; [year of publication].
2. Furukawa TA, Streiner DL, Young LT. Antidepressant and benzodiazepine for major depression (Cochrane Review). In: The Cochrane Library, Issue 4, 2004. Chichester, UK: John Wiley & Sons, Ltd.
3. Jamtvedt G, Young JM, Kristoffersen DT, Thomson O'Brien MA, Oxman AD. Audit and feedback: effects on professional practice and health care outcomes (Cochrane Review). In: The Cochrane Library, Issue 4, 2004. Chichester, UK: John Wiley & Sons, Ltd.
4. The Scottish Office Home and Health Department/Scottish Health Advisory Council, 1994
5. Whicher E, Morrison M, Douglas-Hall P. 'As required' medication regimens for seriously mentally ill people in hospital (Cochrane Review). In: The Cochrane Library, Issue 4, 2004. Chichester, UK: John Wiley & Sons, Ltd.